The
endo
Patient's
SURVIVAL
GUIDE

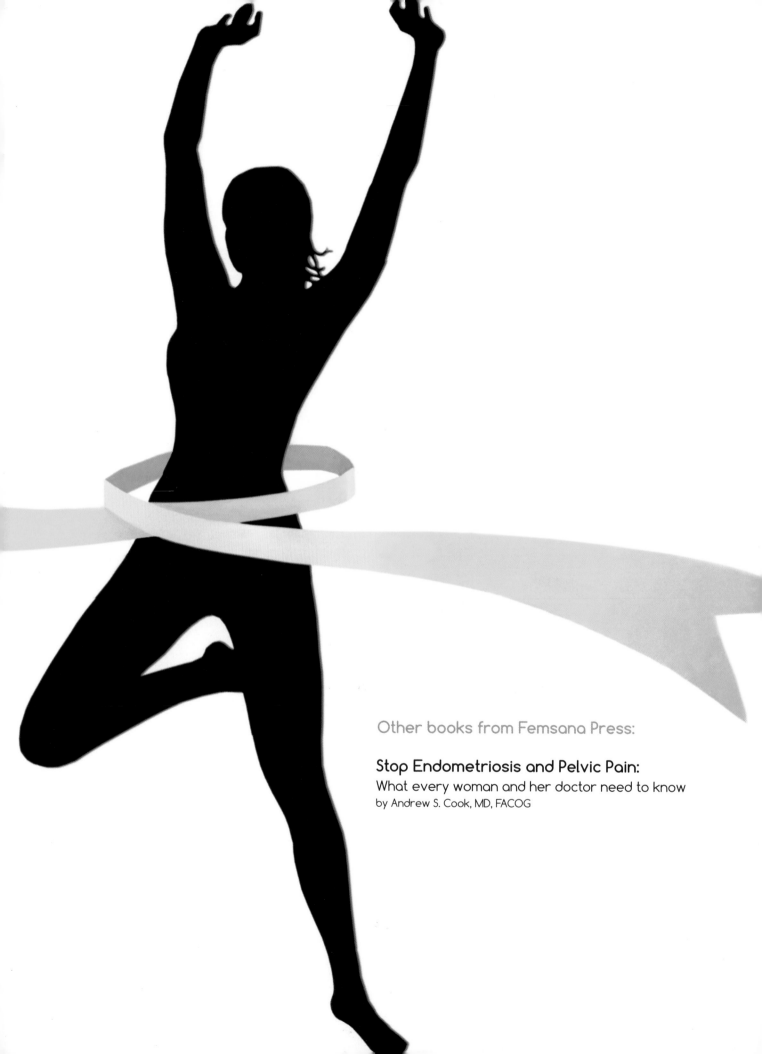

Other books from Femsana Press:

Stop Endometriosis and Pelvic Pain:
What every woman and her doctor need to know
by Andrew S. Cook, MD, FACOG

The
endo
Patient's
SURVIVAL
GUIDE

A Patient's Guide to Endometriosis & Chronic Pelvic Pain

Andrew S. Cook MD, FACOG
Libby Hopton MS
Danielle Cook MS, RD, CDE

Femsana Press
LOS GATOS, CALIFORNIA

Disclaimer

We have made every effort to ensure that the information provided in this guide is accurate and up-to-date. The information provided regarding health and medical treatment is the result of extensive clinical experience with patients as well as reviews of relevant medical and scientific literature. That literature at times reflects conflicting conclusions and opinions, and new research is continually being undertaken. We also involved numerous medical experts as well as patients in reviewing the guide prior to publishing. The reader should understand that there may be a difference of opinion between experts on subjects contained within this guide.

The authors, publisher, and Vital Health Institute specifically disclaim any and all liability arising directly or indirectly from the use or application of any information contained in this book, including third party information referenced in the guide. Information in this publication should not be used as a substitute for professional medical advice or care. The reader should consult a physician in matters relating to her health. In particular, the reader should consult with a competent professional before undertaking any form of self-treatment or acting on any of the information or advice contained in this guide.

References

For a complete listing of the scientific articles and medical textbooks referred to in the production of this guide, please contact libby@vitalhealth.com

Publisher's Cataloging-in-Publication data

Cook, Andrew S.
    The Endo Patient's Survival Guide : A Patient's Guide to Endometriosis & Chronic Pelvic Pain / Andrew S. Cook MD, FACOG , Libby Hopton MS , Danielle Cook MS, RD, CDE.
    pages cm
    ISBN 9780984953516 (pbk)
    ISBN 9780984953523 (e-book)
    Includes bibliographical references and index.

1. Endometriosis. 2. Endometriosis --Treatment. 3. Pelvic pain. 4. Pelvic pain --Treatment. 5. Pelvis --Diseases --Treatment. 6. Menstruation disorders --Treatment. I. Hopton, Libby. II. Cook, Danielle. III. Title.

RG483.E53 C66 2015
618.1 --dc23   2015941747

Printed in the United States of America
10 9 8 7 6 5 4 3 2

We would like to dedicate this guide to each and every woman worldwide who suffers from endometriosis and pelvic pain.

This guide is also dedicated to my mom, Sally Cook, who taught me the true meaning of love and compassion.

Dr. Andrew Cook

Acknowledgments

The content of this guide was co-authored by:

Dr. Andrew S. Cook, MD, FACOG
(Founder & Medical Director of Vital Health Institute)

Libby Hopton, MS
(Director of Research & Evidence-Based Medicine, Vital Health Institute)

Danielle Cook MS, RD, CDE
(Functional Medicine Practitioner, Vital Health Institute)

Reviewers
We would like to thank the patients and colleagues who generously reviewed the guide and provided invaluable feedback.

Editing
Jil Britt, Danielle Cook, David B. Redwine, MD, Margaret Sterner, and Michelle Waterstreet.

Indexing
Indexing by Marla Wilson of Printed Page Productions

Artwork & Photography
Front cover: Natalia Aggiato; page xi: Mario Montagna; pages xii-1: -Marie-; page 2: Ron Leishman; page 4: Hit Toon; page 15: Inna Ogando; page 19: Megastocker; page 25: Bluezace; page 30: Intensem; page 33: Ankomando; pages 42-43: Clker; page 44: Aaaniram; pages 50-51: Clairev; page 52: Mario Montagna; page 65: Diana Barbatti & Kelly Vorves

Artwork, image editing, book design, and layout: Libby Hopton

Funding
This guide was fully funded by Andrew Cook, MD and the Vital Health Institute, Los Gatos, California.

Content

x

Forward

You would think that a condition as common as endometriosis would be well recognized, easily diagnosed, and effectively treated by the medical community, but sadly nothing could be further from the truth. Despite its status as one of the most common conditions affecting womankind, endometriosis continues to elude the medical community at large: women suffer unacceptable diagnostic delays and typically struggle with symptoms for years before receiving an accurate diagnosis. When a diagnosis is finally made, the vast majority of doctors simply lack the knowledge, training, and expertise to adequately treat the disease. The result is a cycle of failed treatments for the patient. Over time and in the absence of effective care, the disease is allowed to wreak havoc on all aspects of a woman's life, robbing her of her vitality, productivity, and happiness.

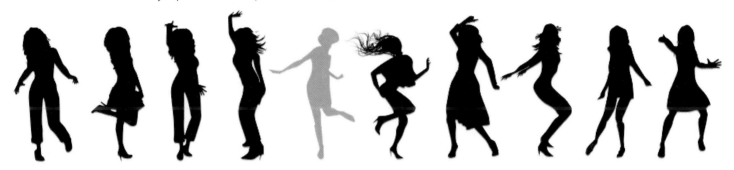

Endometriosis affects 1 in every 10 women, with an estimated 176 million sufferers worldwide

As a specialist who has dedicated his career to improving the care of women with endometriosis, I am confronted by the staggering and debilitating effects of this pervasive disease on women's lives. Through treating thousands of women, I have had the unique opportunity to develop and refine a new paradigm in the effective treatment of endometriosis and pelvic pain; a paradigm that offers hope and restores lives.

This guide is dedicated to each and every woman worldwide who suffers from endometriosis and pelvic pain. My hope is that this resource will serve as a trusted companion on your journey to healing. It contains all the bare essentials needed to help you access optimal care.

I would like to thank all of the women who have entrusted in me their health and who have touched me with their unfaltering strength and courage in the face of this debilitating disease. You have allowed me to learn and develop the expertise needed to successfully treat what is one of the most common yet challenging and humbling conditions affecting girls and women of all ages worldwide.

Andrew S. Cook, MD
Los Gatos, California

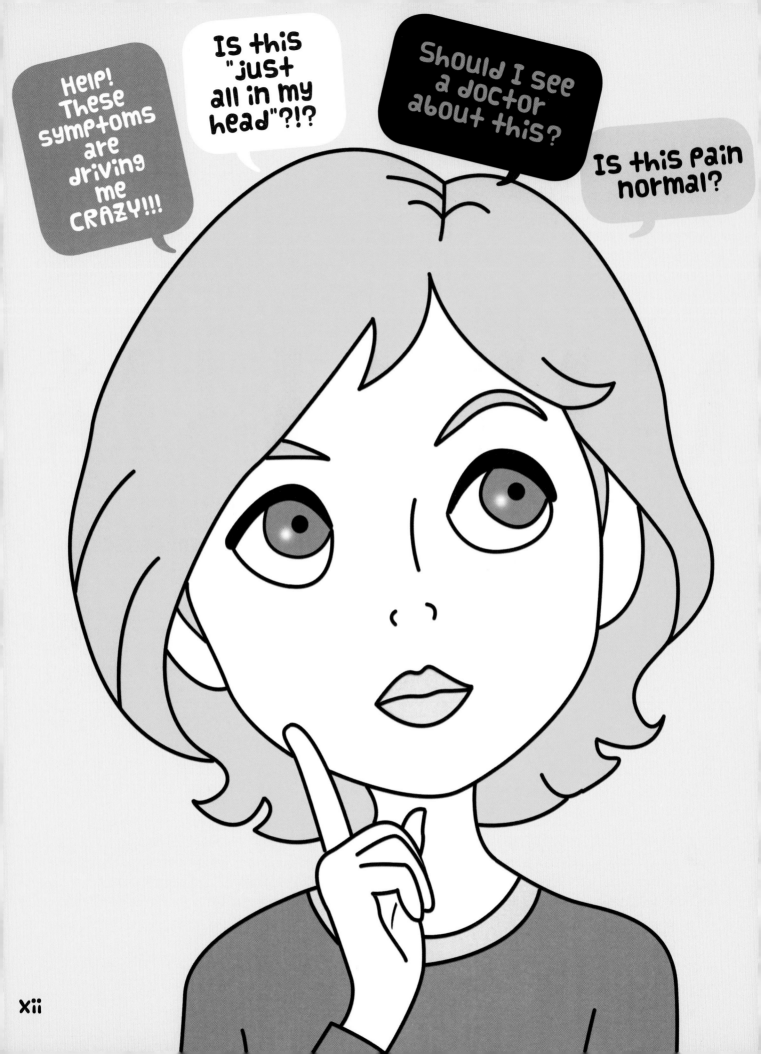

Endo-metri-ermmmmm??? Why couldn't they have given it a simpler name?!

What is endo and how do I know if I have it?

Why does it feel like I just ate a porcupine!?

How is endo diagnosed?

Beginning with the Basics

What are the best treatments for endo?

Is there a cure?

I'm thinking of undergoing surgery. What do I need to know?

What's the cause?

If this isn't endo, what else could it be?

No one seems to understand what I'm going through. How do I find support?

How do I find a specialist?

Is my pelvic pain normal?

Just because something is common does not make it normal. Pelvic pain should be taken seriously. It can point to underlying health problems that can seriously impact your quality of life and, in some cases, can compromise your fertility.

Women who complain about their period pain simply have a low pain tolerance...

NOOOO! The pain associated with endometriosis can be horrific and comparable to the pains of labor. Suffering from debilitating pelvic pain has absolutely nothing to do with your level of pain tolerance.

Every woman has cramps during her period... it's just Mother Nature's monthly wake up call to remind us of our womanhood!

NOOOO! Being debilitated on a monthly basis by severe pelvic pain that does not respond well to pain medications and that prevents you from leading a full and happy life is NOT normal.

It's normal for sex to hurt!

NOOOO! It's not normal to experience pain during or after sex. Sex should be pain-free and enjoyable.

It's normal to have crazy periods during the teenage years. You'll grow out of it...

NOOOO! While irregular periods are common during the first years following menarche, painful periods are never normal, regardless of the girl's or woman's age. One study found that 70% of teenage girls with chronic pelvic pain have endometriosis.

I always suffered from terrible period pain from my very first period. It's just one of those things I have to accept.

NOOOO! Just because something has been affecting your life for a long time does not mean that you just have to live with it. Many women diagnosed with endometriosis have suffered since they were teenagers. The earlier you seek help, the sooner you can get relief.

But my mother, sister, aunt, niece... also have bad period pain, so it must just be normal.

NOOOO! Endometriosis often runs in families and can affect multiple women in the same family. This can lead to the normalization of debilitating pelvic pain and a delay in seeking help. Just because other women you know also happen to have pelvic pain does not mean that it is normal or acceptable. Don't let others invalidate your pain. Educate those around you so they can also seek help.

When to seek help...

Q: Are you experiencing ongoing pelvic pain (chronic or recurrent on a monthly basis) that is interfering with your ability to function or that routinely requires over-the-counter pain medications?

Q: Are you having to plan your life around your pelvic pain? Are you avoiding social engagements and taking time off school or work around the time of your monthly period or when your pain flares?

Q: Are you avoiding sex because it is painful?

If you are experiencing ongoing pelvic pain that is impacting your quality of life, this is **NOT** normal. It is time to seek help.

aaaaaaaaaaaaaaaaaaaaarrrgghhhhhhhhhhh

Tracking your symptoms in 5 easy steps...

Keeping a symptom diary will help you keep track of any triggers or patterns in your symptoms and how they fluctuate or change over time. It can also be an invaluable way of communicating with your doctor about the problems you are experiencing.

1. Daily symptoms

Dedicate a few minutes each day to recording any symptoms you have been experiencing in the past 24 hours.

Make a note of the day in your cycle and then answer the following questions:

Q1: How severe was your pain today from 1 to 10?

Q2: What if anything triggered your pain? (activities, foods, stress, fatigue, and timing in your cycle)?

Q3: Where was your pain located? How would you describe your pain (dull, aching, throbbing, sharp, stabbing, pulling, burning, etc.)?

Q4: Did you experience other symptoms besides pelvic pain (headaches, bloating, flu-symptoms, muscle ache, fatigue, etc.)?

Q5: How did you manage your pain, and did this help (type, dose, and frequency of pain medication use)?

Q6: How did your pain impact your day (avoiding activities, missing school or work)?

2. Menstrual symptoms

Keep track of menstrual patterns: cycle length, heaviness, duration, and any bleeding between periods.

3. Sexual symptoms

Keep track of sexual symptoms: pain during or after sex, the type of pain (pain at the vaginal opening, pain with deep penetration or painful orgasm), bleeding after sex, vaginal dryness, lack of lubrication, and any changes in these symptoms during your menstrual cycle.

4. Urinary symptoms

Keep track of urinary symptoms: pain prior to, during, or after urination, urinary frequency during the day and night, problems emptying the bladder and the presence of blood in the urine. Note any triggers of urinary symptoms.

5. Bowel symptoms

Keep track of bowel symptoms: pain prior to, during, or after bowel movements, bloating, gassiness, nausea, rectal bleeding, and any fluctuations in bowel habits (frequency, urgency, diarrhea, constipation). Note any triggers of bowel symptoms.

Download our symptom diary template at:
www.vitalhealth.com/symptomdiary

Top tips on talking to your doctor about your pelvic pain

The first step to addressing pelvic pain is to acknowledge that something is wrong. The next step is to seek help from your doctor...

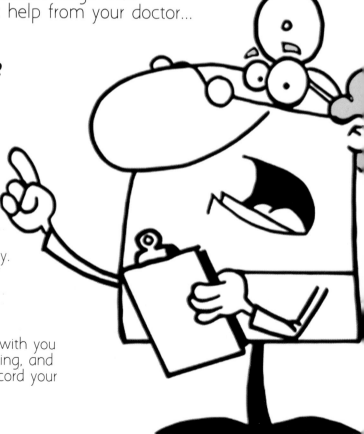

Tip 1
Ensure you have enough time at the appointment

If you feel you will need extra time, ask in advance for a double appointment.

Tip 2
Prepare in advance

Keep a symptom diary, ideally for a month or two prior to your appointment. Prepare a list of questions for the appointment. List them in order of their priority.

Tip 3
Bring a trusted companion

Two sets of ears are better than one. Bring someone with you who can listen, advocate, and support you before, during, and after the appointment. If helpful, ask permission to record your appointment on your phone.

Tip 4
Do not be afraid to speak up

Talk openly about your pain and any other symptoms you are having, including symptoms relating to menstruation, sex, and bowel and bladder function. It can be difficult to discuss these subjects, but your doctor won't be fazed. Talking openly is the only way of bringing the problem out into the open and getting the help you need.

Tip 5
Set goals

If tests or treatments are suggested, discuss a specific timeline for when any results will be discussed, when to reassess the effectiveness of any treatments, and what to do if the proposed treatment does not help.

Make sure that you are happy with any decisions being made. Remember, this is your body, you are an active decision-maker in the patient-doctor relationship. Don't be afraid to question decisions and to ask for clarity if anything is unclear.

Tip 6
When things do not go to plan

If your doctor is unhelpful or dismissive of your pain, take a deep breath and calmly explain the impact your symptoms have on your life. Provide concrete examples.

Second opinion

If your doctor is unhelpful, does not listen, or invalidates your symptoms, you are entitled to a **second opinion** from another doctor.

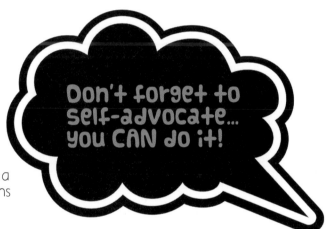

Don't forget to self-advocate... you CAN do it!

Examples:

"Last month I missed a week of work because of severe pain."
"We have stopped having sex because it is too painful."
"I rely on pain medication for most of the month and even then struggle to function with the pain."

If your partner, relative, or friend is with you, have them reiterate what you are saying from their own perspective.

Examples:

"I am having to take time off work to care for the kids because my wife is bedridden for a week each month."
"I am afraid to have sex with my girlfriend because she ends up in tears from the pain."
"We went on vacation together but it coincided with her period, so she ended up spending most of the trip in bed."

Provide your doctor with a copy of your symptom diary.

2. Endometriosis: The Bare Essentials

The Core Medical Facts

Fact: Endometriosis is when tissue that is somewhat similar to the lining of the womb is found outside the womb.

Fact: Endometriosis most commonly involves the peritoneum, which is a thin layer of tissue that cloaks the structures inside the pelvis. Disease that is limited to the peritoneum is referred to as "superficial endometriosis".

Fact: If the disease involves tissue beneath the peritoneum, it is referred to as "deeply infiltrating endometriosis" (DIE) or "deep endo" for short.

Fact: Endometriosis also commonly involves the uterine ligaments, the bladder, the bowels, and the ovaries.

Fact: In very rare cases, endometriosis is found away from the pelvis, involving surgical scars, the diaphragm, and the lung. These rare forms of endometriosis in distant sites are called "extra-pelvic endometriosis".

Fact: Most women with endometriosis have disease that is limited to the peritoneum. Only a minority suffers from deep endometriosis involving the ovaries, the bowel, the bladder, ureters, and other pelvic, extrapelvic, and abdominal structures.

Fact: Women with endometriosis are at an increased risk of: adenomyosis, fibroids, interstitial cystitis, pelvic floor dysfunction, abnormalities of the genitourinary tract, autoimmune disorders (lupus, rheumatoid arthritis, Sjögren's syndrome, and multiple sclerosis), hypothyroidism, chronic fatigue syndrome, fibromyalgia, atopic diseases (asthma and allergies), and certain rare forms of ovarian cancer.

A Closer look at the disease process

Secretory cells
Endometriosis contains cells that secrete chemicals that irritate the tissue inside the pelvis.

Inflammatory immune response
The immune system detects these chemicals and this triggers ongoing inflammation. As a result, blood capillaries local to areas of endometriosis may swell, burst, and bleed. Over time, scar tissue may form as a result of the irritants being secreted and from the associated inflammation they cause.

Scarring and adhesions
If scarring is severe, it can start to fuse adjacent tissue and organs together (pelvic adhesions).

Pain and infertility
The secretory chemicals, the associated inflammation and the presence of scarring and adhesions can all cause debilitating pain and other symptoms, including infertility in some patients. Symptoms vary, depending on where the endometriosis is located and on how active the glands are. Hormonal changes during the menstrual cycle often affect the activity of the glands, and, in turn, the severity of symptoms.

Disease ≠ Pain
Disease severity does not predict pain severity. Superficial endometriosis and deep endometriosis alike can be excruciatingly painful and debilitating. Conversely, some patients remain largely symptom-free despite the disease.

Cause

We do not know the cause of endometriosis, although several theories of origin have been proposed. It is likely that multiple causal pathways involving interacting developmental, genetic, epigenetic, and environmental factors contribute to a woman's risk of having endometriosis, the severity of her symptoms, and how extensive the disease ultimately is.

Endo runs in families
Multiple genes have been linked with endometriosis. The disease often runs in families. If your mother or sister has the disease, you are at an increased risk of also receiving the diagnosis.

Endometriosis is neither contagious nor infectious!

Symptoms

Common symptoms of endometriosis

✱ Cyclical pelvic pain (pain that worsens just prior to and during menstruation and/or during ovulation)
✱ Non-cyclical pelvic pain
✱ Deep pain during sexual intercourse
✱ Pain during bowel movements, especially during menstruation
✱ Cyclical rectal bleeding

Note: Not all patients will present with all of these symptoms. The nature of a patient's symptoms will depend on where her disease is located and whether other coexisting conditions are present. Symptoms may vary or worsen over time.

Common symptoms in women with endometriosis, which may or may not be directly related to the condition

✱ Intestinal cramping, bloating, and cycles of constipation and diarrhea
✱ Pain on emptying the bladder and with fullness of the bladder
✱ Urinary frequency during the day and night, difficulties emptying the bladder, blood in the urine, and flank pain
✱ Uterine cramping and heavy menstrual periods
✱ Lower back and leg pain during menstruation
✱ Pain during orgasm
✱ Fatigue
✱ Infertility

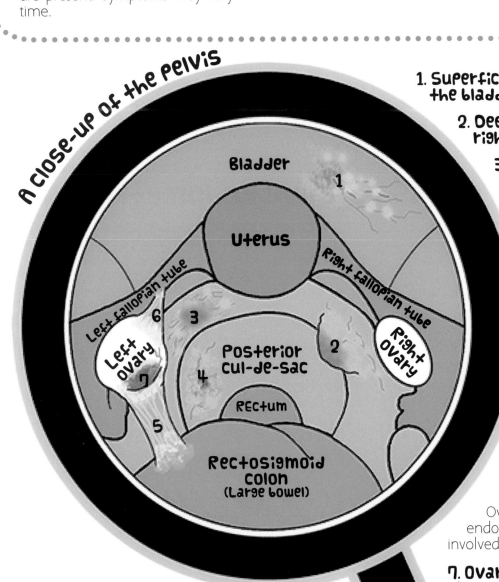

A close-up of the pelvis

1. Superficial endometriosis of the bladder

2. Deep endometriosis of the right uterosacral ligament

3. Superficial endometriosis of the left uterosacral ligament

4. Superficial endometriosis of the posterior cul-de-sac

The most common sites of endometriosis are the posterior cul-de-sac (the space between the uterus and the large bowel) and the uterosacral ligaments (the bands that connect the uterus to the lower back).

5 & 6. Adhesions (scar tissue) involving the left ovary.

Ovaries containing endometriomas are often involved by adhesions.

7. Ovarian endometrioma (chocolate cyst).

Ovarian endometriosis is associated with pelvic disease elsewhere and a higher risk of intestinal endometriosis.

Endometriosis can vary from mild to severe. The location, size and depth of lesions vary widely between patients.

7

Could I have endometriosis?

I'm just a teenager. Am I too young to have endometriosis?

NOOOO! The youngest reported case of symptomatic endometriosis was in an 8 year old girl who had not yet started her period. Endometriosis is a leading cause of pelvic pain in teenage girls.

I've already had children, can I still have endometriosis?

YES! Pregnancy does not cure endometriosis. Having had children does not rule out this diagnosis.

Can the symptoms of endometriosis persist following natural, medical, or surgical menopause?

YES! While symptoms often lessen post-menopause, some patients continue to experience endometriosis-related pain.

I have painful periods. Does that guarantee that I have endometriosis?

NOOOO! While endometriosis is a leading cause of pelvic pain, it is not the only cause. For example, uterine cramping is often caused by diseases of the womb such as fibroids and adenomyosis.

I have endometriosis. Does that mean that my daughter will also develop the disease?

NOT NECESSARILY. While daughters of mothers with endometriosis are at an increased risk of also being diagnosed with the disease, the majority of first-degree relatives of endometriosis sufferers do not have endometriosis. It is best to remain vigilant about any symptoms you recognize in your daughter and support her in seeking help, if and when she needs it.

What it really means to have endometriosis...

Quite frankly, a lot of this medical-talk can be quite dry and boring and does not convey what it is like for a woman to have this disease and how it truly impacts her life, her family, her career, her sex life, and her ability to live her life in very basic ways.

> In reality, this disease can be like having tens or hundreds of excruciatingly painful blisters covering the inside of the pelvis.

Patients with endometriosis can experience horrific pain. For the lucky ones, it lasts just a couple of days during their period, but in the worst cases the pain is 24/7. The dichotomy between the way women with endometriosis look well on the outside but are experiencing excruciating pain internally can cause even well-meaning people to doubt the severity of their pain.

Most women begin to have pain in their teenage years, sometimes even starting in junior high school. While similar in timing, this pain is completely different than normal menstrual cramps.

It is not uncommon for these girls to miss a couple of days of school each month from cyclic pain that can exceed the level of pain patients experience after major surgery.

A lack of awareness of this disease can leave these girls without a correct diagnosis and support from their physicians. This can lead to a lack of appropriate treatment for the pain and invalidation of the patient's situation. Her family is now led to believe that psychological issues drive the severity of her pain.

> In this tragic situation, she is effectively held prisoner and tortured by her own body in broad daylight, with no one who fully understands her situation or who can effectively help her.

The symptoms usually progress as she matures into a young woman. Both the severity and duration of the pain typically increase. Initially, most days each month are pain-free, but the number of these days slowly decreases until there are a greater number of non-functioning pain days. The unpredictability of the increasing number of pain days makes it challenging to maintain a functional life.

It becomes increasingly difficult to make plans for a future date, as it becomes more likely that it will be a pain day, and she will not be able to follow through on her commitment to the activity.

As a disease, endometriosis can take away many additional aspects of a normal life. Mothers cannot reliably meet the needs of their children when the pain is too severe to function. Wives try to push through the pain to be intimate with their husbands, but eventually the pain becomes too intense to continue. Grinding fatigue, as severe as that experienced with advanced cancer, is present in many cases. Bloating, moodiness, and bladder and bowel issues are common as well.

Feeling like a vibrant desirable woman is long since gone. Acting like the loving, compassionate woman, mother, and partner that she truly is becomes more and more difficult. The stress on family relationships is common and real.

Even at this stage, most women fight the disease, refusing to let it completely take over their life. You would most likely pass right by them in public, having no idea of the devastation they are dealing with. Most of the time they get up, put on a brave face, and do their best to live a normal life.

It's time to break the taboos and change attitudes so that no woman need suffer in silence.

3. Diagnosing Endometriosis

How is endometriosis diagnosed?

When evaluating for possible endometriosis, your doctor will usually conduct the following assessments...

1. Medical history
Your doctor will start by reviewing your medical history and will ask you about the symptoms you have been experiencing. Taking your symptom diary along with you to your appointment can be a helpful way of communicating about your symptoms.

Endometriosis has an average diagnostic delay of 7-10 years.

2. Pelvic exam & Pelvic Pain Mapping
Your doctor will perform a pelvic exam. During the exam, not only the size and motility of the uterus and ovaries will be assessed, but also the tissue behind the uterus will be palpated, as this is the location where endometriosis is most commonly found. Tenderness and nodularity in this area is highly suspicious of endometriosis. An important technique in assessing for possible endometriosis is pelvic pain mapping. This is where the doctor maps out any areas of tenderness by carefully touching the posterior cul-de-sac with the fingertips during a digital vaginal exam. This may be uncomfortable but can provide valuable information about the source of your pelvic pain.

Careful evaluation by an experienced doctor is necessary for a timely diagnosis.

3. Ultrasound
Your doctor may perform a transvaginal ultrasound. The ultrasound wand is carefully inserted vaginally, and the pelvic organs are imaged, including the uterus, ovaries, bladder, and rectosigmoid colon (the last section of large bowel). An ultrasound can detect ovarian endometriomas (chocolate cysts) and can sometimes detect deep endometriosis involving the bowel and posterior cul-de-sac. It will not however detect superficial disease, which is the most common type of endometriosis.

4. Diagnostic laparoscopy

If your doctor suspects endometriosis, a diagnostic laparoscopy may be advised. This is a minimally invasive surgical procedure performed under general anesthesia. The doctor first inflates your pelvis with CO_2 gas and then inspects the pelvic structures via a laparoscope, a viewing tube with a small camera attached, inserted through a small incision in your belly button. Additional incisions may be made near each hip bone to allow more surgical instruments to be introduced. Laparoscopy is often called belly button surgery because of the small incisions. A special instrument called a uterine manipulator is also placed through the cervix and into your uterus. This allows the surgeon to move the uterus forward in order to view the areas most commonly affected by endometriosis.

A doctor who performs a diagnostic laparoscopy to diagnose endometriosis should be familiar with the subtle visual appearances of endometriosis and should examine the pelvic surfaces closely enough not to miss any disease. If areas of visually abnormal tissue are found, they should be removed, and the specimens sent to a pathologist for biopsy confirmation. Biopsy confirmation is the gold standard in diagnosing endometriosis.

Note: Not all surgeons are equally experienced in making this assessment, and sometimes the disease can be missed. Finding a surgeon who specializes in the surgical treatment of endometriosis is preferable. It is helpful to request that your surgeon takes photos during your surgery, and ideally a video, so that you have a copy in your medical records. This way, if there is any doubt about the surgical findings, you can easily seek a second opinion and have your records reviewed.

My scan came back normal... does that mean I don't have endo?

NOOOO! If your scan comes back normal, this does NOT exclude the possibility of endometriosis. Scans (ultrasound, MRI, and CT) can be helpful in detecting ovarian endometriomas (chocolate cysts) and deep endometriosis. While ovarian cysts are easy to detect, detecting deep disease depends on the skill and experience of the professional who interprets the images. Superficial endometriosis and adhesions are not usually seen on scans. The best way to assess whether you have endometriosis is during diagnostic laparoscopy.

Can Lupron diagnose endo?

NOOOO! Sometimes patients are erroneously told that the drug Lupron can be taken to "diagnose" endometriosis. The rationale is that if the patient responds, her pain must be hormone-related and, therefore, endometriosis. The problem with this line of logic is that 1) not all women with endometriosis experience symptom relief while on Lupron, and 2) symptom relief may occur for a number of hormone-mediated gynecological conditions while on this drug.

SO... responding to Lupron does not guarantee that you have endometriosis and failing to respond does not exclude endometriosis as a possible diagnosis. For this reason, use of Lupron to "diagnose" endometriosis is controversial.

Differential diagnosis

It isn't uncommon for a woman with endometriosis to be misdiagnosed with various other conditions before the correct diagnosis is made. This is because 1) there is no non-invasive test for endometriosis, and 2) some of the symptoms of endometriosis are also associated with other common conditions.

Common misdiagnoses
Irritable bowel syndrome (IBS)
Pelvic inflammatory disease (PID)
Acute appendicitis
"Your pain is all in your head!"

Multifactorial pain

It is not uncommon for a patient to have multifactorial pelvic pain (the pain has more than one cause). Endometriosis may be just one of several factors in a woman's pelvic pain. Common conditions that co-exist with endometriosis include:

Adenomyosis
Fibroids
Interstitial cystitis (IC)
Pelvic floor dysfunction (PFD)
Adhesion-related disorders

Sometimes endometriosis can overshadow other sources of pain, including acute appendicitis, which represents a medical emergency.

If my pelvic pain is not due to endometriosis, what else might it be?

Here are some of the most common causes of chronic pelvic pain...

Uterus
* **Adenomyosis:** Endometrial-like tissue found within the muscular uterine walls can cause severe menstrual cramping, heavy, prolonged menstrual flows, deep pain during intercourse, and painful orgasm.
* **Fibroids:** Benign uterine tumors made of smooth muscle tissue can cause heavy, painful menstrual flows, pelvic pressure, and pain.

Bladder
* **Interstitial Cystitis (IC):** This chronic condition of the bladder can cause lower pelvic pain, urinary frequency and urgency, and pain when the bladder is full.

Bowel
* **Reduced bowel motility, redundant colon, food sensitivities & intolerance:** These gastrointestinal problems can cause IBS-like symptoms.
* **Bowel obstruction:** A small bowel obstruction can cause pain, nausea, and vomiting. A large bowel obstruction can cause pain, constipation, and diarrhea.

Adhesions
* **Adhesion-related disorders:** Adhesions and scar tissue resulting from disease, infection, injury, or surgery can constrict or stretch pelvic structures, causing pain, infertility, and bowel obstruction.

Ovary
* **Ovarian cysts:** Ovarian cysts, if persistent, may stretch the ovary, causing lower right- or left-sided pelvic pain. Cyst rupture can cause severe pain.

Appendix
* **Chronic appendicitis:** Chronic inflammation of the appendix can cause right-sided pelvic pain.

Vulva
* **Vulvodynia:** The vulva (the tissue around the vaginal opening) can be a source of pain.

Pelvic floor
* **Pelvic floor dysfunction:** Over-tightening of the pelvic floor muscles can cause pelvic pain, such as pain with bowel movements, urination, and sexual intercourse.

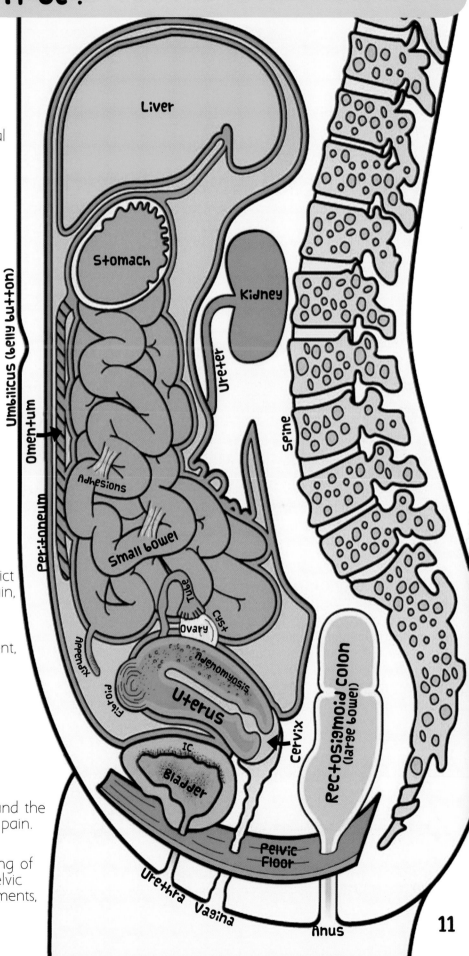

11

4. Coping with Endometriosis

Building a network of support

There are girls and women all around the world and from every walk of life who are coping with endometriosis. **You are not alone.** Reaching out to the patient community can be a great way of building a network of support.

Communicating about endometriosis with others...

What do I tell others?

Firstly, you don't have to say anything. Talk about endometriosis on your terms, when you feel comfortable to do so. What you tell someone in any given situation will depend on your relationship with them, their reason for asking, and how you are feeling at the time. Even at the best of times, endometriosis isn't the easiest condition to explain to others. Therefore, having some printed educational materials (such as this guide) on hand to share at home, school, or work can be a great way of educating others about your condition.

Connect with your national patient organization: Endometriosis.org/support/support-groups

Unwanted advice

When someone is in difficulty, it's natural to want to help by offering some advice. Sometimes, that advice may be based on misinformation. **"Why don't you just get a hysterectomy. My aunt's son's best friend's sister did that and feels great now!"** Often the best way to respond is to simply say **"Thank you, but each individual case is different."** Again, if you feel up to it, these can be great opportunities to educate others by sharing accurate printed materials that state the facts.

Asking for help

Don't be afraid to ask help from others. Having friends and trusted family members to help in times of need can make a huge difference. This can be anything from helping around the house and offering childcare and/or pet-sitting, to accompanying you to doctor appointments, and being there for you when you have surgery, or simply offering a listening ear during difficult times.

When loved ones don't understand

Sadly, friends, partners, and family members may not always be as understanding as they should be. Many struggle to understand that:

* someone can be so severely debilitated by an invisible disease **"But you don't look sick!"**
* some illnesses may not get better over time or fully resolve following surgery **"Are you still sick? I thought you had surgery?"**
* some symptoms may be associated with and, therefore, confused with normal bodily processes **"So basically you're just having period pains?!"**

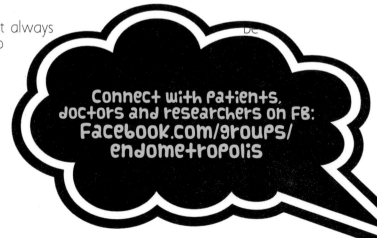

Connect with patients, doctors and researchers on FB: Facebook.com/groups/endometropolis

Simple ways of helping those around you to understand...

1. Education: Provide accurate, authoritative information for friends and family to read and process in their own time. **Vitalhealth.com** contains lots of easy-to-read resources for just this purpose.

2. Involvement in care: Invite them to your doctor visits, so they can ask any questions they may have.

3. Support groups: Invite them to attend a patient support group meeting or suggest they join an on-line support group, where friends and family are welcome.

4. Articulate your needs: Tell them how they can help, even if it may seem obvious: **"Mom, I just want you to be there for me. I know you can't fix this and it's difficult to see me in pain, but a hug and someone to talk to would go a very long way right now."**

5. Be patient: When loved ones first hear of your diagnosis, it can take time for them to come to terms with this. Often parents, loved ones, and friends go through phases of shock, denial, anger, disbelief, and confusion before finally acknowledging and accepting the truth and being there for you. Giving others time to come around, rather than burning bridges, can be the best strategy in the long run, albeit difficult short term.

6. Communicate: Being open and communicating your needs and feelings candidly is an essential means of allowing those close to you to understand and to be there for you. People take many things for granted in life; women with endometriosis often put on a brave smile despite the amount of pain they are in. Sometimes, simply explaining the impact of this disease on your daily life (what you can do, what you cannot do, and how you feel physically and emotionally) can help others understand how debilitating this condition is for you.

7. Professional help: Sometimes communication and education are not enough. In such situations, family therapy and/or couples counseling may provide valuable lifelines to patients and their loved ones. This can aid in coming to terms with the impact of endometriosis, not only on the patient but on the whole family unit.

Coping with BAD PAIN DAYS

Seeking urgent help for pain

* If in doubt, check it out! If your pain is severe and/or accompanied by nausea and fever, get checked out by your doctor or go to urgent care or the emergency room. Endometriosis can sometimes mask other potentially life-threatening conditions that may require urgent medical care.

* Analyze your symptoms: Try to analyze your symptoms in terms of location and type (uterine, bladder, bowel, and vaginal). While endometriosis may be the first source that comes to mind, reflect on other possible factors that might be contributing to your pain. Consider possible bladder infection, appendicitis, yeast and bacterial infection, tummy trouble, or constipation. Disentangling the symptoms and possible causes can be helpful when deciding what course of action to take.

* Go prepared: Prepare well for an ER or doctor visit. Take someone with you if at all possible. If a planned visit, prepare any questions you have, written down on paper. Take a diary of your symptoms and what you have tried until now to deal with them. Try to stay calm. Be persistent when seeking help. It is easy to get flustered. If you feel that way, take a deep breath, pause, and try again to convey your message and what you need. If heading to the ER, have a folder on hand (best to keep this ready if ER visits are common) with all your essential medical information. This will enable the staff to easily assess what treatments you have had. Be clear as to what you are hoping to achieve and which symptoms are particularly worrying you. Set your priorities.

* Right to care: Don't leave the ER until you are comfortable doing so. The staff have an obligation to help you, and you have a right to receive care.

Coping with pain at home

* Anticipate the flare: Keep a pain diary to establish any patterns in your pain. This can help you predict when the pain will likely be worse, so you can prepare for, or even keep ahead of it, by taking pain medication before the pain strikes. Keeping on top of your pain is ideal if possible. Discuss your pain flares with your doctor, so that together you can find a good strategy to deal with them. Have an agreement on when it is time to seek extra help and when to manage the pain at home. Specialist pain management might be required.

* Pain medication: Take pain medication before the pain begins or as soon as you can feel the pain coming on. This will help you stay on top of the pain, and may actually reduce the amount of medication needed to manage your pain. This is especially important when recovering from surgery. Just remember, to minimize withdrawal symptoms, taper off of pain medications gradually.

* Beauty Sleep: Severe pain can interfere with sleep. If you find that your pain medications wear off during the night, consider setting your alarm clock mid-way through the night so you can wake up and take more pain meds. This will help you keep on top of your pain until the morning.

* Muscle relaxers: Pain medication can be combined with muscle relaxants for increased relief (discuss this first with your doctor).

* Take care of yourself: Don't neglect other vital aspects of your heath when in pain. Don't forget to drink, eat, and get enough sleep.

* Heat and Ice: Try using a heating pad (be careful not to fall asleep with it on, and be careful not to burn yourself) and/or an ice bag to soothe painful areas.

* Zen: Create a calm, soothing home environment: play soft music, light scented candles (pleasant scents have been found to improve pain tolerance), put on comfy clothes, turn the heating up, dim the lighting, and snuggle up with a nice soft blanket.

* Soothing Oils: Apply castor oil or lavender essential oil (externally) to your pelvic area. **Warning:** caster oil can cause a skin reaction. First test a small area of skin before applying to a larger area.

* Soaking in the tub: Take a long hot bath (consider using lavender Epsom salts).

* Meditate, visualize, and relax: Use visualization to escape to a calm place. Practice deep breathing or follow a guided meditation.

* A soothing massage: Ask your partner, a close friend, or family member to give you a gentle, relaxing massage.

* Bend like a banana: Elevate the legs and upper body with cushions, forming an arc-shape with your pelvis at the bottom. You could also lie in a hammock.

* Not the fetal position: Try to avoid curling up in the fetal position as this will only cause your muscles to tense, which may add to your pain.

* A glass of wine: A glass of wine or ginger beer can be relaxing, although for some, alcohol causes their pain to flare. **Note:** alcohol should not be consumed in combination with certain medications. Check first!

* Rocking chair: Rock back and forth in a rocking chair.

* A healing dose of humor: Having a laugh might be the last thing you feel like when in pain, but it has been found to help both as a distraction and as a way of improving pain tolerance. Being around positive, friendly, smiling people may make you feel a little bit better. In contrast, best to avoid negative people and potentially negative interactions while in pain.

* Something to swear by: When going through a painful experience, off-setting the pain with some curse words has actually been found to help. So, if you feel like it, let it all out. It may just help!

* The power of distraction: If your pain is not too severe, distracting yourself with something enjoyable may help take your mind off of it. For example, lose yourself in a good book (or audiobook), watch a film, play a game, or go for a brisk walk or run. Obviously, adapt the activity to something that you feel like doing and that falls within your comfort level.

* Gentle exercise and stretching: For mild pain, gentle stretches, Pilates, yoga, and Tai Chai may help (you may want to seek the advice of a physical therapist if you are seeing one).

* Food for thought: Adjust your diet according to your symptoms. If you find that you have problems with your bowels at the time of your period, such as constipation and rectal pain, adjust your diet to try and minimize the constipation or take stool softeners (if used frequently, discuss with your doctor). Cut down on sugar and other pro-inflammatory foods. Seeking the advice of a dietitian who works with women with endo may help. For more information about diet, see page 44.

* Think Positive: Severe pain is sometimes accompanied by feelings of depression. If you are feeling "down" as well as in pain, try to set yourself a goal, something to look forward to, or work toward. For example, decorating a room, looking through old photos, going out shopping or taking a spa day. Try not to dwell on the losses associated with this disease, but rather savor the happy times, the successes, and the triumphs despite all you are going through. You are an endo warrior not an endo worrier. Don't let this disease defeat or define you.

5. Treating Endometriosis

Weighing up your treatment options

Once you have a (suspected) diagnosis of endometriosis you will find yourself at a crossroad, with different treatment options that can potentially lead to very different outcomes. Even your choice of doctor can play a critical role in how your endometriosis is treated. The decisions you make now can have long-term consequences for your health. For this reason, taking the time to research your options, considering the pros and cons of each type of treatment, asking your doctor any questions you may have, and if needed, seeking a second or third opinion, are all important steps in ensuring that you receive the very best of care. **Become informed and self-advocate!**

How to make informed decisions about treatment

In order to make informed decisions about your care, you need to know about all treatment options available, including their risks (side effects, complications, and any potential implications on fertility and other health factors) as well as their benefits (success rate, expected symptom relief, and how long-term any relief is expected to last).

Your doctor should provide you with all of this information, but this may not happen because:
* The doctor lacks sufficient knowledge about current treatment options and so only offers limited or outdated information.
* The doctor has not maintained data on his/her patient outcomes following treatment so cannot provide accurate information about expected outcomes and complication rates.
* The doctor discusses treatments he or she feels comfortable offering and does not mention treatments that could otherwise benefit the patient but would require referral to a specialist.
* There is not enough time scheduled to go over all of your options.

Ask your doctor questions about treatment outcomes and treatment options. Do your own research, and seek a second opinion if you don't feel you've been adequately informed.

Your role in decision-making

As the patient, you are at the center of your healthcare team and play a critical role in any decisions made about your treatment. It is your body and ultimately your choice of which treatments you undergo. If you feel like you are being pushed into a treatment you do not feel happy about, discuss this openly with your doctor. If needed, take the time to seek a second opinion to see if other options are available.

Realistic expectations

When going into any treatment, it's important to have realistic expectations. While no treatment offers 100% success, most women with endometriosis can expect considerable, ongoing relief of their symptoms with the right treatment. This may mean combining different treatments and/or seeking the help of a doctor with specialized expertise in treating endometriosis.

Some women with endometriosis have multi-factorial pelvic pain and other health problems. In these patients, endometriosis is not the only cause of their symptoms. Therefore, other coexisting conditions may need to be diagnosed and treated to provide optimal relief.

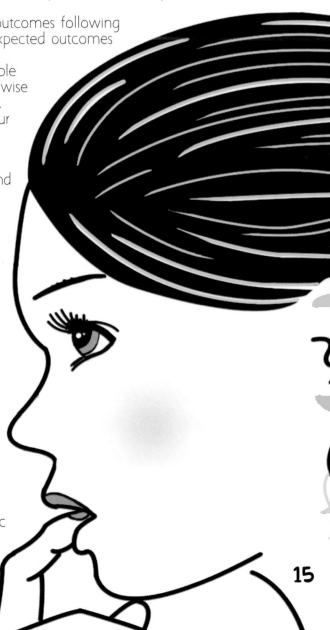

15

How is endometriosis treated?

The treatments you will be offered will depend on:

* **Symptoms:** depending on whether you are seeking treatment for pain and/or infertility

* **Disease severity:** the type and severity of your condition (superficial disease, deep disease and/or cystic ovarian disease)

* **Surgical skill:** the surgical skill and experience level of the doctor treating you

* **Your preferences:** your personal wishes and circumstances

* **Medical history:** maybe you have already tried certain treatments previously or perhaps certain treatments are contraindicated (unsafe) because of certain health, family, and lifestyle factors

There are 3 approaches to treating endometriosis:

5.1 Medical therapy (treating the symptoms)

5.2 Surgical treatment (treating the disease)

5.3 Comprehensive multi-system approach (improving and maintaining over all health)

5.1 Medical Therapy

Hormone therapy

What does hormone therapy do?
Hormone therapy suppresses the production of hormones by the ovaries.

How does hormone therapy help relieve endometriosis-related pain?
Endometriosis contains estrogen receptors that respond to estrogen released by the ovaries. Estrogen can affect the activity of endometriosis. By reducing estrogen levels, the hope is to reduce disease activity and in turn reduce your pain.

How effective is hormone therapy in relieving endometriosis-related pain?
Hormone therapy has been found to provide some relief in at least 75% of patients. However, it may not provide complete relief, and many patients experience side effects that can be difficult to tolerate.

Can hormone therapy treat endometriosis-related infertility?
No, hormone therapy used to manage endometriosis is not suitable for patients who are trying to conceive, and It does not improve fertility.

Will hormone therapy make my endometriosis shrink or go away?
No, hormone therapy at best reduces symptoms associated with endometriosis and other hormone-mediated conditions. It does not make endometriosis go away, and the effects stop soon after you stop taking the medication.

What types of hormone therapy are available?

Combined hormone therapy:

Combined hormone therapy suppresses ovarian function and contains low doses of estrogen and progesterone. The effect is to lower the levels of estrogen. There are many types of combined hormone therapy on the market. Most are taken orally (the pill), but non-oral variants are also available.

Common side effects include:

Breakthrough bleeding, breast tenderness, bloating, headaches, mood changes, decreased libido, and changes in appetite.

Progesterone-only hormone therapy:

Progesterone-only hormone therapy works in a similar way to combined hormone therapy but only contains progesterone. Progesterone-only hormone therapy can be taken orally (the mini-pill), via an injectable depo that is released over time, or via an intrauterine device (IUD) that is inserted through the cervix into the uterus.

Common side effects include:

Breakthrough bleeding, breast tenderness, headaches, fatigue, nausea, mood changes, bloating, and weight gain.

Testosterone-like hormone therapy (Danazol):

Danazol works by suppressing the signals in the brain that make the ovaries produce estrogen. Danazol is taken orally (pill form) containing a testosterone-like hormone.

Common side effects include:

Breakthrough bleeding, weight gain, bloating, acne, increase in body hair, decrease in breast size, and deepening of the voice (which may be a permanent side effect).

Gonadotropin-Releasing Hormone Analogues (such as Lupron):

GnRH-a therapies, such as Lupron and Zoladex, work by suppressing ovarian hormone production by acting on the pituitary gland. Unlike other hormone therapies, GnRH-a therapies do not contain hormones. For this reason, they induce a state of medical menopause. GnRH-a therapies are administered via nasal spray or injection.

Common side effects include:

Menstrual irregularities, hot flashes, vaginal dryness, decreased libido, insomnia, thinning of the bones, mood changes, acne, and joint pain.

Aromatase inhibitors:

Aromatase inhibitors work by inhibiting the enzyme (Aromatase) that synthesizes estrogen. The main source of estrogen in the body comes from the ovaries, but secondary sources include fatty tissue as well as endometriotic tissue. Aromatase inhibitors stop all synthesis of estrogen.

Common side effects include:

Menstrual irregularities, hot flashes, vaginal dryness, decreased libido, thinning of the bones, mood changes, and joint pain.

Coping with side effects

Will I get side effects?

While side effects are common with hormone therapy, each woman responds differently. Some women experience a lot of side effects that make the treatment difficult to tolerate, while others experience few, if any, side effects.

What can I do about side effects?

If worrying side effects develop, discuss them with your doctor. If taking hormone therapy daily, make sure you take the dose at the same time each day. Certain side effects may decline over time. You may want to persevere for a while to see if things improve. If the side effects don't improve, changing to a different hormone therapy or a different dose may help. In the case of GnRH-a therapies, taking add-back therapy (small doses of estrogen or progesterone) may help reduce some of the menopausal side effects.

Hormone therapy... continued

If I do not respond to hormone therapy, does that mean my pain is not due to endometriosis?

No, not all women with endometriosis experience improvement while undergoing hormone therapy.

Which hormone therapy is best?

Studies comparing hormone therapies have not found one particular type to be more effective than the others. Finding the best hormone therapy for you is individualized and may take some trial and error.

Is hormone therapy for me?

While some women find hormone therapy to be very helpful in reducing their pelvic pain, other women find they develop intolerable side effects, or hormone therapy is simply not helpful. In some cases hormone therapy is not indicated because the patient's medical history places her at risk of serious side effects.

If I'm not on hormone therapy, will my endo get worse?

Many patients will experience progression of their symptoms over time. Hormone therapy has neither been found to prevent progression nor recurrence of endometriosis.

Pain Management

Adequate pain management is paramount in women with endometriosis, because of the chronic and debilitating nature of this painful condition.

The type of treatments offered will depend on the type of pain, its severity and duration, and your specific needs and wishes. The goal of pain management is to bring your pain under control so that you can function.

Pain management is often a short-term strategy to provide relief until you can access treatments that offer lasting improvement. In some cases, however, ongoing pain management in the form of prescription and non-prescription drugs and interventional pain management may be required. Long-term pain management is typically overseen by a pain management physician who communicates with others on your medical team.

Non-prescription pain medications

Non-prescription pain medications commonly used to manage pelvic pain include Acetaminophen (Tylenol) and non-steroidal anti-inflammatory drugs (NSAIDS) such as Ibuprofen and Naproxen. NSAIDS inhibit the release of prostaglandins and suppress inflammation. They are most effective when taken before your pain sets in and should be taken with food.

Care needs to be taken not to exceed safe daily doses of pain medication, especially when combining different non-prescription and prescription drugs. It is important for your safety that even over-the-counter medications are disclosed and carefully discussed with your doctor when considering pain management options.

Prescription pain medications

Prescribed pain medications include prescription NSAIDS and narcotics. Narcotics can be short acting (such as hydrocodone, oxycodone, and hydromorphone) or long acting (such as morphine and long-acting oxycodone). Narcotic pain medications work by slowing down or stopping the signals from the nerves to the brain. The choice of narcotics prescribed will depend on whether your pain is acute (such as post-operative pain) or chronic (ongoing pain).

> **Do NOT combine prescription and non-prescription pain medications without consulting your doctor!**

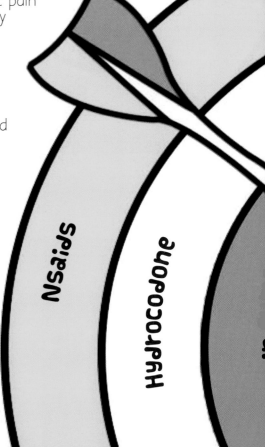

NSaids

Hydrocodone

Pain-Narcotic Contract

If you receive prescription-narcotic pain management, you may be required to enter into a pain-narcotic contract. This contract specifies what you can and cannot do while taking prescription-narcotic pain medications. The pain-narcotic contract is in place to ensure your safety while taking these medications.

Interventional pain management treatments

Interventional pain management treatments for long-term pain include: pain pumps (an implantable pain-management device), spinal cord stimulators (pain catheters), trigger-point injections or nerve blocks (temporary numbing injections of painful areas or overly sensitive nerves), and radiofrequency ablation (RFA), where targeted nerves are "stunned." RFA offers more prolonged relief than nerve blocks.

Dependence & Addiction

There's a social stigma around taking narcotics. Many patients are worried they'll become addicted. But there's an important difference between physical dependence and addiction.

Dependence: If you stop taking the drug suddenly you experience physical withdrawal symptoms, such as flu-like symptoms. Dependence is common with prolonged use of narcotics, but can be resolved by tapering off of the drug gradually.

Addiction: Addiction is when you crave a drug and engage in compulsive drug-seeking and drug-misuse despite harmful effects. In patients with no prior addiction issues, the likelihood of problems with addiction to the narcotics taken for pain is very low.

If you are in severe pain, you need and deserve effective pain relief, and sometimes that means taking narcotics.

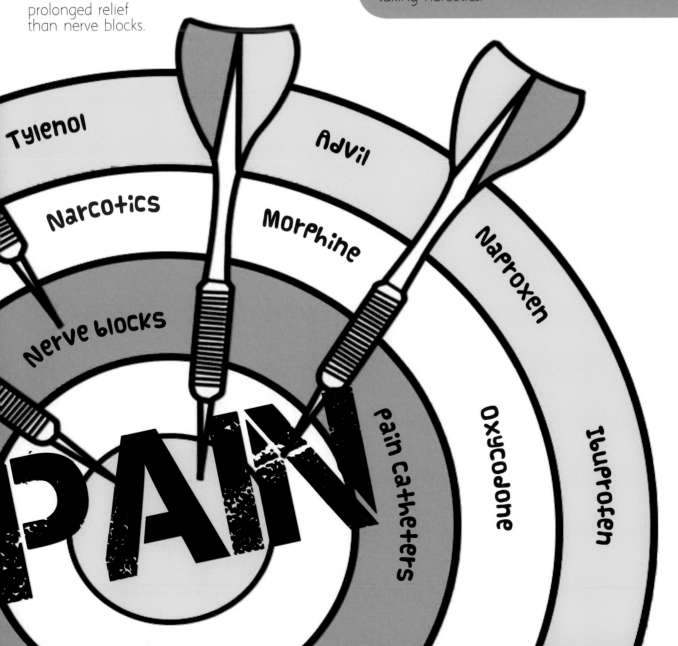

Surgical treatment

Surgical treatment is the only treatment for endometriosis that has been proven to eradicate the disease from the body.

Goals of endometriosis surgery
* Identify all areas of endometriosis inside the body
* Eradicate and/or remove all areas of endometriosis
* Divide any adhesions
* Provide ongoing relief of endometriosis-related pain
* Improve fertility (if endometriosis is a cause of infertility)

Types of endometriosis surgery
* "Belly-button" surgery (traditional laparoscopy or robotic laparoscopy)
* Open surgery (laparotomy)

Benefits of laparoscopic surgery over laparotomy:
* Lower risk of post-operative adhesions (less scarring)
* Smaller incision size
* Lower risk of infection
* Better illumination and visualization of the areas of endometriosis
* Shorter hospital stay and a quicker recovery

Is open surgery ever necessary?
Nowadays, even the most complex of endometriosis surgeries are being performed successfully via laparoscopy. The more experienced and skilled the surgeon, the more able he or she will be to conduct complex procedures via laparoscopy rather than having to revert to open surgery. Under certain exceptional circumstances, however, open surgery may be required.

* In cases of very severe adhesions (such as in patients who have had multiple previous laparotomies), laparoscopy may be too difficult, risky, and/or time consuming.
* If endometriosis surgery is being combined with removal of a very enlarged uterus (such as in the case of multiple, large fibroids) open surgery may be inevitable.
* If a segment of bowel is severely involved by endometriosis and needs to be removed, the surgeon may perform a mini-laparotomy. This is where one of the small incisions is extended slightly in length to allow a section of bowel to be passed outside the body.
* Very rarely, a complication may occur during surgery, requiring the surgeon to convert from laparoscopy to open surgery to address the problem quickly.

Open surgery is often advised in cases where the surgeon does not have the necessary expertise to perform the same procedure via laparoscopy. By seeking a second opinion from a more experienced surgeon you may be able to avoid the need for open surgery.

Surgical incisions

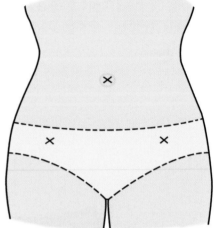

Traditional laparoscopy

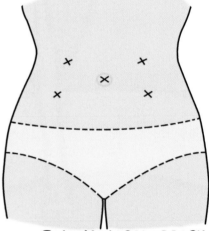

Robotic laparoscopy

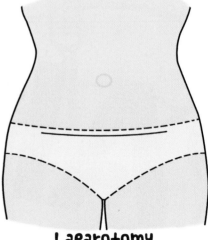

Laparotomy

What happens during laparoscopic surgery?

1. After you are given a general anesthetic to put you to sleep, a catheter is inserted into your bladder to empty it.

2. A pelvic exam is performed and a uterine manipulator is inserted into the uterus. The uterine manipulator enables the surgeon to adjust the position of the uterus, enabling complete visualization of the pelvic cavity during surgery.

3. The abdominal cavity is insufflated (inflated) with CO_2 gas introduced through a hollow needle. The gas provides more space within the pelvis, enabling visualization during surgery.

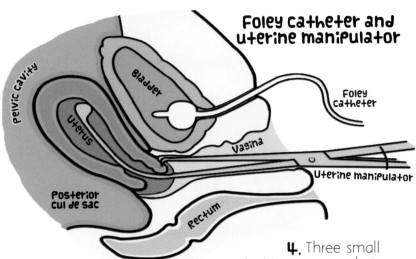

Foley catheter and uterine manipulator

Pelvic cavity

Bladder

Uterus

Foley catheter

Vagina

Uterine manipulator

Posterior cul de sac

Rectum

4. Three small incisions are made in the pelvic area: one through the belly button (umbilicus) and two beneath the bikini line. A trocar (cylindrical sheath) is placed through each incision. The laparoscope, a thin fiber-optic tube with a camera attached, is inserted through the umbilical trocar and connected to large video monitors. This enables the surgeon to inspect the inside of the pelvis. Surgical instruments (such as the laser, irrigator, and graspers) are placed through each of the trocars.

Digital Processing unit

Biopsy tray

Assisting Surgeon

Laser unit

Anesthesia unit

Video monitor

Laser & Laparoscope

Patient

Assistant

Anesthesiologist

Instrument tray

Surgeon

Bird's eye view of the operating room

5. Using the graspers and the laparoscope, the surgeon carefully inspects the pelvic and abdominal surfaces for any areas of endometriosis. All areas of visually abnormal tissue are then treated and biopsies are removed from the body and sent to the pathologist.

6. Once surgery is complete, the surgical instruments are removed, the abdomen is deflated, the incisions are closed, and you are taken to recovery. The catheter may be left in place until you are well enough to get up and use the restroom.

Cross-sectional view

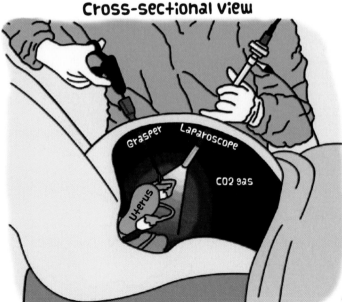

Grasper

Laparoscope

CO_2 gas

Uterus

Surgical techniques - what's the big deal?

The choice of surgical techniques is critical to the success of your surgery
While there are many different tools being used by surgeons to treat endometriosis, ultimately it's not the tool that matters, but rather the technique which that tool is used to perform.

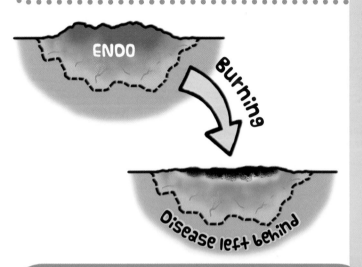

Burning

Also known as:
Coagulation, fulguration, diathermy, and cauterization.

What happens to the tissue?
A low-energy heat source is used to disrupt the tissue. With burning, the heat spreads throughout a large area, potentially damaging healthy tissue. A recent study found that burning techniques leave endometriosis behind in 80-90% of cases.

When should this technique be used?
The only time when this technique should be used is to control bleeding (hemostasis). It should NOT be used to treat endometriosis.

Excision

Also known as:
Linear vaporization

What happens to the tissue?
Either mechanical energy (scissors) or a high-energy heat source (such as laser and electrosurgery) is used to cut out the diseased tissue, leaving only healthy tissue behind. When excising using energy, the heat is concentrated on a small area of tissue only. This minimizes damage to surrounding healthy tissue.

When should this technique be used?
Excision is the mainstay of endometriosis surgery and should be used in ALL but exceptional situations (**99%** of the time).

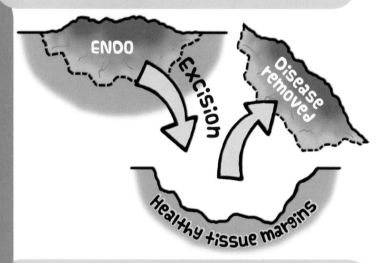

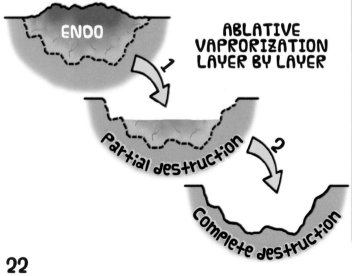

ABLATIVE VAPORIZATION LAYER BY LAYER

Ablative vaporization

Also known as:
Area vaporization

What happens to the tissue?
A high-energy heat source is used to transform a small area of tissue into vapor. When vaporizing, the thermal energy is concentrated to a small area of tissue only. This minimizes damage to surrounding healthy tissue. The diseased tissue is destroyed layer by layer.

When should this technique be used?
Ablative vaporization is reserved for exceptional situations (**1%** of the time) where excision would otherwise compromise fertility or potentially increase risk of complications.

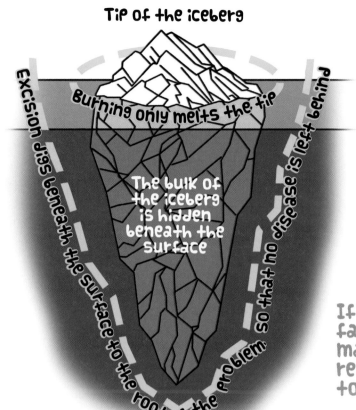

Tip of the iceberg

Burning only melts the tip

The bulk of the iceberg is hidden beneath the surface

Excision digs beneath the surface to the root of the problem, so that no disease is left behind

Why is burning best avoided?

Burning is not a reliable method of eradicating endometriosis. It does not provide a biopsy of the diseased tissue, it cannot be applied to diffuse areas of disease, and it cannot be safely applied to disease overlying vital structures.

Burning endometriosis is akin to melting the tip of an iceberg. While it may look like the disease has been fully treated, the bulk of the disease is often left behind and just beneath the surface.

If the surgical technique used fails to eradicate the disease you may well experience persistence or recurrence of your pain and have to undergo further surgery.

Is excision always best?

Excision is an effective means of removing all areas of endometriosis and providing biopsies of diseased tissue. It can be safely and effectively applied to more or less any area of tissue in the body. For this reason, excision is the best surgical technique when treating endometriosis... **BUT**.... in a limited number of situations layer-by-layer ablative vaporization can provide a valuable alternative to excision. One such example is treatment of superficial endometriosis on the surface of the ovaries.

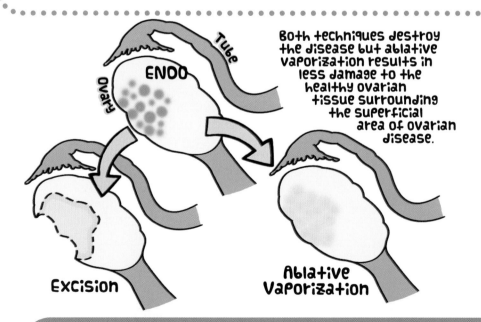

Tube

Ovary

ENDO

Both techniques destroy the disease but ablative vaporization results in less damage to the healthy ovarian tissue surrounding the superficial area of ovarian disease.

Excision

Ablative Vaporization

Endometriosis on the surface of the ovaries:

While excision could be used to treat superficial endometriosis of the ovary, it is less precise than ablative vaporization and could lead to unnecessary loss of healthy ovarian tissue, potentially compromising the patient's fertility.

The disadvantage of ablative vaporization is that it does not provide a biopsy of the treated tissue and only small areas can be reliably treated.

Watch real examples of endometriosis surgery:
www.vitalhealth.com/videos

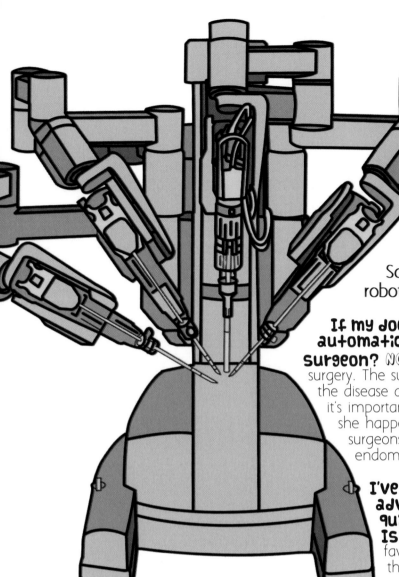

What's the verdict on robotic surgery?

The rise of robotic laparoscopy has enabled more surgeons to perform a wider range of minimally invasive gynecological surgery (in place of open surgery) than ever before. The learning curve involved in performing surgery via the robot is considered to be less steep than with traditional laparoscopy. So what, if any, advantages does the robot offer in the treatment of endo?

If my doctor uses the robot, does that automatically make him/her a good endo surgeon? NOOOO, the robot is just a tool used to facilitate surgery. The surgeon still needs to know how to recognize the disease and how best to treat it. So, first and foremost, it's important to choose the surgeon not the tool that he/she happens to use. There are excellent endometriosis surgeons who use the robot, just as there are excellent endometriosis surgeons who use traditional laparoscopy.

I've heard that the robot is more advanced and that recovery is quicker than with other types of surgery. Is that true? While the robot compares favorably to open surgery (which is rarely used in the treatment of endometriosis), it is no more advanced, no quicker, nor safer than traditional laparoscopy. It actually typically involves more incisions that are more noticeable (above the bikini line) than the incisions used for non-robotic laparoscopy. Recovery times and surgical outcomes are also comparable between these two forms of surgery. The robot may, however, aid in providing 3D visualization of affected tissues (although 3D vision is now also available via traditional laparoscopy), more intuitive controls (making it easier for trainee surgeons to learn to operate and allowing greater articulation of the surgical instruments), and a more comfortable operating position for the surgeon (which may be advantageous during longer cases). It's unclear at this point, however, as to whether these features translate into superior clinical outcomes in patients with endometriosis. More research is needed. Conversely, robotic surgery lacks the tactile (haptic) feedback of traditional laparoscopy, which could make it more difficult for the surgeon to differentiate between healthy and abnormal tissue, especially when treating deep disease. Given that the same set of surgical principles apply, regardless of whether a surgeon performs surgery robotically or via traditional laparoscopy, at the end of the day, it is the surgeon's expertise and skill that is of greatest importance.

Is robotic surgery more dangerous than traditional laparoscopy?

NOOOO, while all surgery carries risks, robotic surgery is no more risky than traditional laparoscopy. Again, the greatest determining factor in risk of complications is the surgical skill of the surgeon performing the surgery. The robot does not replace a need for skill and adequate training.

In summary...

Pros:
* 3D vision
* Easier to learn than traditional laparoscopy
* More comfortable for the surgeon

Cons:
* Less cosmetic (more incisions that are more visible than traditional laparoscopy)
* No haptic (tactile) feedback

Conclusion: The robot is a tool that may aid surgery but has **NOT** been shown to provide superior outcomes over traditional laparoscopy.

Finding an endometriosis surgeon

Choosing the right surgeon can make the difference between undergoing an effective surgery that removes all of your disease and undergoing an ineffective surgery where disease is left behind and symptoms persist or recur. For the best outcome, it is important to find a surgeon who has the necessary expertise to remove ALL of your endometriosis.

Why does endometriosis surgery require a high degree of expertise?

Endometriosis comes in many visual presentations. It takes considerable experience to recognize and remove all forms of this disease. In advanced cases of endometriosis, the disease involves multiple organ systems, and the pelvic anatomy is distorted by dense adhesions (scar tissue) that bind organs together. Only the most experienced and skilled surgeons can successfully treat advanced forms of endometriosis.

What happens if my surgeon is not skilled enough to do my surgery?

A surgeon who lacks the expertise needed to treat endometriosis may fail to recognize all areas of disease. Some areas may intentionally be left untreated through concern about damaging vital structures. If the disease is not fully removed, the surgeon may suggest other treatments, such as hormone therapy and pain management. Lack of expertise can result in a patient entering an ongoing cycle of surgeries without resolution of her symptoms.

Is removal of my uterus and ovaries a good alternative to removal of the disease?

Said simply, no. Sometimes, if a surgeon is unable to remove the disease, he or she will recommend the patient undergo a hysterectomy (with retention or removal of her ovaries) to "treat" her endometriosis. Removing the uterus will **ONLY** treat uterine pain (pain coming from the uterus due to another condition and **NOT** pain caused by your endometriosis). If your pain is primarily caused by endometriosis, hysterectomy is very unlikely to help (as it does not remove the disease) and will render you unable to carry a baby. Removing the ovaries may potentially relieve pelvic pain in some women with endometriosis **BUT** will place you into an immediate state of surgical menopause. This could well replace one set of symptoms with a whole new set of symptoms with further-reaching implications on your health. Therefore, endometriosis should be treated by removing the disease, not removing healthy reproductive organs (the uterus and ovaries). Certain pelvic conditions other than endometriosis may, however, require hysterectomy and, in exceptional cases, removal of one or both ovaries as a last resort.

In an ideal world the disease should be removed and the woman's reproductive organs should be preserved where possible. In the vast majority of women with endo, radical surgery can and should be avoided. Too many patients have been pushed into parting with their reproductive organs without realizing other surgical options are both available and effective.

Questions to ask a Prospective Surgeon...

1) Surigcal technique: What type of surgery do you do? What techniques do you use? When would you perform excision and under what circumstances might other techniques be used instead? What proportion of the surgery will be performed via excision? What are the benefits of the specific techniques you use? Are you able to perform my surgery laparoscopically?

2) Experience: How long have you been doing endometriosis surgery and how many cases have you done? Do you perform these surgeries on a weekly basis?

3) Expected outcomes: What is the prognosis regarding pain relief, disease recurrence, and fertility in my case? What can I expect based on the outcomes you have had with previous patients with a similar presentation of the disease?

4) Scope of surgical treatment: Do you treat both deep and superficial endometriosis? Can you remove the disease from all areas? What if the disease involves my bowel, bladder, ureters or diaphragm? If not, will surgeons from other specialties be on hand to assist?

5) Approach to bowel disease: If bowel disease is present, how do you treat it? Do you have surgical privileges to perform bowel surgery? Under what circumstances would a bowel resection be performed? Would this be performed laparoscopically? What are your complication rates with bowel surgery? What are your views on bowel surgery (more conservative such as, "avoid resection if possible," "resection is rarely needed," or more radical such as, "resection is generally needed if invasive bowel disease is present"?

6) Preserving organs: Will my organs be preserved? Under what circumstances would an organ be removed?

7) Preventing adhesions: What do you do to prevent/reduce the risk of adhesions? What success have you had with these approaches?

8) Risks & complications: What are the risks involved in undergoing this surgery? What are your complication rates? How often do you convert from laparoscopy to laparotomy?

9) Biopsy confirmation: Will all areas of disease that are removed during surgery be sent to a pathologist for histological diagnosis? If not, why not?

10) Chief surgeon: Will you be doing my surgery? (Perhaps an odd question but in some settings the actual surgery may be undertaken by a colleague or junior surgeon, possibly under supervision).

11) Persistent pain: What if my pain recurs/persists despite this surgery? Will you continue to support me and offer me treatment? What other treatments do you have to offer besides surgery?

12) Post-operative pain management: What kind of post-operative pain management will I receive? What if this is insufficient?

13) Post-operative follow-up: What kind of post-operative follow-up care will I receive?

14) Traveling for care: What provisions are there in place for patients traveling long-distance for surgery? How will I keep in touch after surgery should I have any problems?

15) Assistance with insurance: How much experience does your office have in assisting me with the process of obtaining insurance coverage and can you work with me to help me afford the surgery?

16) Case review: Can you review my case from a distance (phone consult and record review)?

For some of these questions, there might not be a "right" or "wrong" answer. Knowing your surgeon's take on the matter can help you make an informed decision as to whether this is the surgery you want and to form accurate expectations about the likely outcome of the surgery.

Common myths about endometriosis surgery

For a patient to make informed decisions about surgery, she needs accurate information. Unfortunately, many healthcare professionals are not up-to-date on the latest clinical research on endometriosis. While well-meaning, they may inadvertently provide inaccurate information. This can lead to uninformed and sometimes life-changing patient decisions and can prevent women with endometriosis from accessing optimal surgical care.

Ovarian suppression (such as with Lupron) will make surgery easier

NOOOO! Hormone therapy does not make the disease shrink or go away. It may make the disease harder to spot, increasing the risk of incomplete surgery (disease left behind).

Hysterectomy will cure your endo!

NOOOO! Hysterectomy (removal of the uterus) neither cures nor treats endo. This treatment option should be reserved for patients who have a problem with the uterus itself (such as uncontrolled heavy bleeding and/or uterine pain).

Removing your ovaries will cure your endo!

NOOOO! While removing the ovaries may relieve the symptoms of endometriosis in some patients, it does not remove the disease and it will place you into immediate surgical menopause, which is associated with debilitating symptoms and increased health risks. Less radical treatments can provide relief without causing early menopause.

Pregnancy will cure your endo!

NOOOO! While pregnancy may reduce symptoms in some women with endometriosis, symptoms typically return soon after giving birth and/or weaning. There are many women with symptomatic endometriosis who have previously been pregnant.

Surgery to remove your disease will make you infertile

NOOOO! Actually, research shows that excision of endometriosis can improve fertility outcomes. Even in cases of extensive ovarian endometriosis, a skilled surgeon can almost always remove the disease while preserving your reproductive organs and fertility. Removing your endo does NOT necessitate removing your reproductive organs!

Surgery to remove your endo is too dangerous!

NOOOO! While one surgeon may not be able to surgically treat your endo, this does not mean that no surgeon can. The skill of the surgeon determines the complexity of surgery he or she can offer. If in doubt, seek out a second opinion with a more experienced surgeon.

Excision surgery is a bad idea, as it will cause lots of adhesions

NOOOO! While any surgery can cause scarring, there is no evidence that excision causes more scarring than other surgical techniques. Most patients undergoing excision surgery do not require reoperation for adhesions.

I can only remove what I can see. Invisible disease will be left behind

NOOOO! As long as the disease is recognized in all its subtle forms, it can be removed completely via wide excision, with no disease left behind.

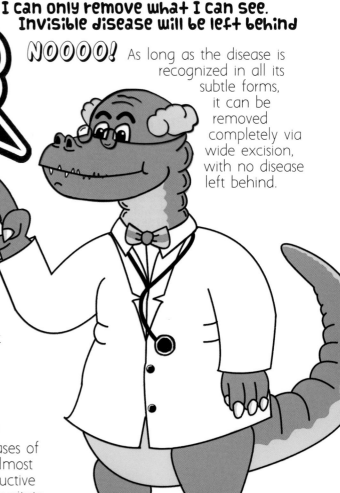

Trust me I'm a gynesaurus!*

*A doctor who relies on myths, not science, when treating patients with endometriosis.

Disease recurrence and persistence after surgery

When patients experience recurrence of their pain and disease weeks, months or years after surgery to treat endometriosis, the conclusion is usually that the disease is "back" and that it "always comes back". However, true recurrence of endometriosis following complete excision is actually very rare...

My pain is back... therefore my disease must be back... right?!

NOT NECESSARILY!!! Recurrence of pain does not necessarily mean recurrence of endometriosis. Pelvic pain is often multi-factorial in nature (having more than one cause). Just because pain persists or recurs despite surgery does not per se mean that your disease is back. Disease recurrence/persistence is just one possible explanation for recurrent or persistent pain despite surgery. Either way, it is important that your pain is investigated and addressed.

Dr. Cook's surgical results

Dr. Cook has operated on thousands of women with endometriosis and has been following up on his patients for over a decade. The results show that with thorough, wide excision of all areas of visually abnormal tissue, the vast majority of patients do not experience disease persistence or recurrence and do not require further surgery for endometriosis. In cases where disease has persisted/recurred, the amount of disease is almost always minimal.

what's the difference between disease recurrence and disease persistence?

Disease recurrence is when new disease forms after the surgery, usually in locations where the disease had not previously been documented. Recurrence is extremely rare (one such example is endo forming at the site of a previous surgical incision).

Disease persistence is when disease is missed or incompletely treated during surgery and so persists (remains) where it is and may continue to cause pain (or cause recurrent pain further down the line).

Disease may persist after surgery for a variety of reasons:

✱ Subtle disease may simply be overlooked, especially if the surgeon is not familiar with the many visual appearances of endometriosis.
✱ Some surgical techniques often fail to fully destroy the disease, leaving diseased tissue behind.
✱ If excision is not wide enough or deep enough, some disease may be left behind.
✱ Sometimes areas of disease are left behind intentionally, because the surgeon is concerned about damaging vital structures, or may lack the expertise to treat that particular area of the body.
✱ Hormone therapy at the time of or just prior to surgery may hinder the visual detection of all areas of disease, causing subtle disease to be missed.
✱ Sometimes "new" disease appears to have formed between 2 consecutive surgeries, but often what has really happened is that subtle disease has become less subtle in appearance over time, and so is more readily detectable during the later surgery.

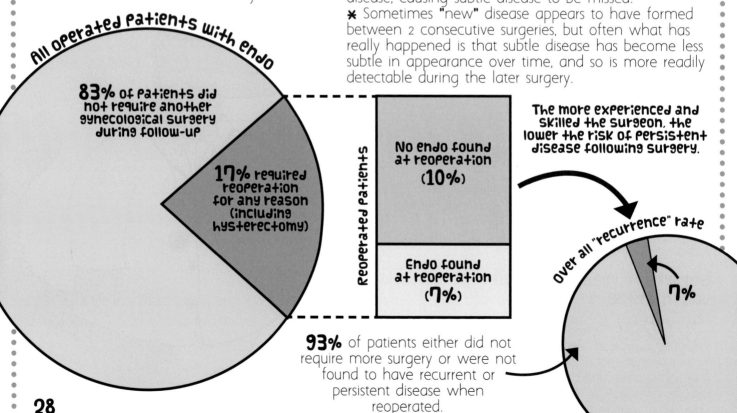

All operated patients with endo

83% of patients did not require another gynecological surgery during follow-up

17% required reoperation for any reason (including hysterectomy)

Reoperated patients

No endo found at reoperation **(10%)**

Endo found at reoperation **(7%)**

The more experienced and skilled the surgeon, the lower the risk of persistent disease following surgery.

Over all "recurrence" rate

7%

93% of patients either did not require more surgery or were not found to have recurrent or persistent disease when reoperated.

The great debate: Can surgery cure my endo?

NO IT CAN'T!!!

YES IT CAN!!!

But the disease ALWAYS comes back!

No it doesn't! If surgery is incomplete then some disease is left behind and may continue to cause pain. BUT if the correct surgical technique is used (wide excision of all affected areas), the disease RARELY recurs, and most patients can expect a future free of endometriosis. They're cured. While endometriosis cannot be prevented, it can be cured!

Wait a minute! What about invisible microscopic disease that the surgeon cannot see and therefore cannot remove?

While surgeons are humans and humans make errors, endometriosis is not an invisible disease. If the surgeon has sufficient experience to identify the disease in all its subtle appearances and uses wide margins when excising the tissue, then the disease can be completely removed.

So you're telling me that with the right surgery, my pain will be "cured" forever?

Well, not quite. Pelvic pain can have many causes. Only if the pain is due to endometriosis will removal of the endometriosis provide ongoing resolution of that pain, in most cases, and that means undergoing the correct type of surgery. If the pain has another cause, you may need other treatments to resolve or manage that. It is true that a lot of women with endometriosis also have other health problems, so physically removing the disease may be just one step toward overall recovery. Another important point is that many women are not offered the necessary surgery to remove all of their disease.

Hmmm... I still don't want to call this a curable disease given that, even with the disease gone, I may continue to have pain from other related pelvic conditions, such as adhesions, interstitial cystitis, pelvic floor dysfunction, and adenomyosis. That doesn't feel like a cure to me! Calling it a "cure" feels invalidating... even insulting to me!

Well, that's a good point, and that's why this is a tricky topic. At the end of the day, each individual has to think of her condition in a way that she feels best represents her reality and experience with the disease. She might think of her condition as chronic, cured, or perhaps in remission. But the important point is that removing the disease fully is both effective and necessary to bring about the best outcomes, and in most cases, the disease does not recur after complete removal. For this reason, it would be a great step forward if all women could access the specialized surgery needed to actually remove the disease.

Well, I guess I can't argue with that!

Phew!

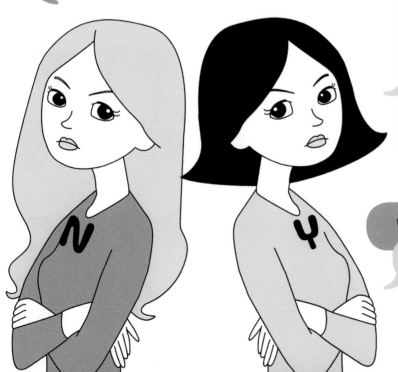

The ins and outs of bowel preparation...

The purpose of pre-operative bowel preparation is to cleanse your intestinal tract, so that it can be safely operated on. While this process is unpleasant to endure, it is necessary in minimizing the risk of complications during bowel surgery.

There are several bowel preparations on the market. Some involve drinking large volumes of laxative drink, while others combine a single laxative drink with an enema solution or oral tablets. The prep may be combined with a low fiber diet during the days that precede it. On the day of the prep (the day before surgery) you will be required to follow a strict diet of clear liquids only. Whichever method you are given, be sure to **follow all instructions carefully!**

Top tips on getting through a bowel prep:

✱ Eat lightly the days prior to the prep. This should make cleansing your intestines a little easier.

✱ Some patients find the prep drink difficult to palate because of the unpleasant taste. Allowing it to cool in the fridge, or packing it in ice in the sink, may make the drink a little bit more palatable.

✱ Try sucking on a Popsicle to cool your tongue just prior to taking a gulp of the prep.

✱ Drinking the prep through a straw can help reduce contact with your taste buds as the liquid passes through your mouth.

✱ If you feel nauseated, try alternating between a pleasant tasting liquid, such as broth, clear fruit juice, or ginger ale, and the prep. Ginger can help with nausea. Try sipping ginger ale or sucking on hard ginger candy. Another trick is to compensate and counteract the unpleasant taste with something pleasant smelling, such as scented candles or a handkerchief sprayed with your favorite perfume. Lavender scents are good against nausea and can help boost pain tolerance (such as intestinal cramps).

✱ To get the unpleasant taste out of your mouth, follow-up the prep drink with something pleasant tasting such as broth, a hard candy, or chewing gum (but be sure to keep to the dietary instructions provided by your physician).

✱ Be sure to remain hydrated during the prep. Drink plenty of clear fluids throughout.

✱ Once the cleansing process begins, use wet wipes instead of regular toilet paper. If you get sore from wiping, apply topical non-prescription hemorrhoid cream, which contains a local anesthetic and will numb the area.

✱ Once the prep begins to take effect, you may start to experience intestinal cramping. Applying a heat pad or ice pack may help soothe this pain.

✱ Provide yourself with pleasant distractions, such as reading materials, portable music player, a film to watch, and entertaining apps for your phone or tablet to tide you over during the prep.

✱ Lastly, remind yourself that many have gone before you, and that this is the last hurdle before a surgery that will hopefully provide you with ongoing relief from your pain. **YOU CAN DO IT!!!**

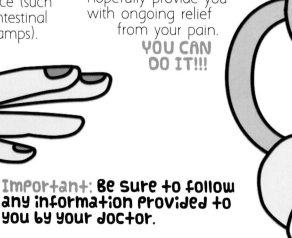

Oh no!!!

Important: Be sure to follow any information provided to you by your doctor.

Things to arrange BEFORE surgery

✳ Time off work: Arrange sufficient time off work to recuperate. This will depend on the extent of surgery, your physical condition, and the nature of your work. It may be best to ease back into activities gradually. If possible, first work half-days before resuming full-time work.

✳ Pets & Kids: If you have young children and/or pets, arrange for a trusted person to help care for them during your first week following surgery. Do not lift your children and/or pets during your recovery!

✳ Housekeeping: Make sure the house is clean and any chores are done BEFORE surgery, so that you don't have to worry about that when you get home.

✳ Groceries: Make sure your kitchen is stocked with food so that you don't have to do a grocery run just after getting home (carrying heavy shopping bags should be avoided during your recovery).

✳ Accompanying Person: If at all possible, arrange for someone to accompany and advocate for you during your hospital stay.

✳ Post-op medications: Request and fill your post-operative pain medications BEFORE surgery.

✳ Clothing: After surgery, your abdomen may feel swollen and tender. Your regular clothing may feel tight and uncomfortable. Make sure you have some wireless bras and oversized underwear/sweat pants (preferably with a wide loose-fitting waistband). Loose-fitting dresses may be more comfy than pants.

Items for the hospital bag

✳ Clothing: Loose-fitting underwear, over-sized yoga/sweat pants, wireless bra, slip-on shoes, bathrobe, and a nightgown.

✳ Toiletries: Toothbrush, toothpaste, hairbrush, chapStick, saline nasal spray, hand lotion, pantyliners, and pads.

✳ Electronics/entertainment: Cell phone, phone charger, kindle or iPad with eBooks/games, and crossword puzzles.

✳ Paperwork: Hospital address, surgeon's name and contact details, surgery documents, health insurance details, contact details of the person who will collect you from the hospital after discharge, and your hotel address and contact details (if traveling for surgery).

What to expect after surgery

✳ Gas Pain: The CO_2 gas used during surgery often causes temporary shoulder pain. Keeping active (light walking) and drinking mint tea will help disperse the gas. Keeping on top of pain medications will help control your pain.

✳ Bowel symptoms: Gassiness, bloating, constipation, and intestinal cramping are common symptoms following surgery. Be sure to drink plenty of non-carbonated, non-alcoholic, caffeine-free beverages during the first days following surgery. Also, stick to soft, bland, nutritious foods that are easy on your stomach and low in fiber. Gas-X can help reduce gassiness and bloating, and bowel softeners and laxatives can help against constipation.

✳ Vaginal bleeding: Light to moderate vaginal bleeding is common for the first few days following surgery. Be sure to have pantyliners and pads on hand to protect your underwear.

✳ Cycle irregularities: Surgery can disrupt your cycle causing your period to come earlier or later than usual.

✳ Fatigue: It is normal to tire more easily during the first weeks following surgery. Ease back into daily activities gradually, and don't overdo it!

Painful menstruation post-op

The first 1-3 menstrual flows post-op may be unusually painful. This can be discouraging and may lead you to question whether the surgery has been successful. Try not to panic. Painful periods are common during the initial healing process. You may initially require additional pain management. This pain should improve as your body heals.

When to call your doctor...

Contact your doctor immediately if any of the following symptoms occur:

✳ High fever (over 100°F)
✳ Uncontrollable pain
✳ Rapid heart rate (120 BPM)
✳ Vomiting or severe nausea
✳ Excessive vaginal bleeding
✳ Rectal bleeding
✳ Pain/swelling in the feet or legs
✳ Pain, urgency and/or frequency of urination, or blood in the urine
✳ Coughing, shortness of breath, or chest pain
✳ Redness, swelling, pain, bleeding, or discharge at the incision sites.

Comprehensive Multi-System Approach

What is a whole-person approach?

There is more to endometriosis than the lesions of pelvic disease. First, the disease often co-occurs with other health conditions (**evil siblings of endometriosis**) that perhaps share common underlying environmental, genetic, and epigenetic risk factors. Second, the chronic pain and inflammation caused by endometriosis may in turn set off a chain reaction that can affect a person's overall health and wellbeing (**domino effects of endometriosis**).

For this reason, treatments that solely focus on relieving specific symptoms and/or removing the lesions may not be sufficient to fully restore overall health. A combination of therapies may be required to address dysfunction across multiple systems within the body.

A whole-person approach considers all aspects of a person's health rather than focusing on a single symptom or a single disease process.

What is multi-systemic dysfunction?

In Western medicine, we traditionally think of individual diseases having specific symptoms, resulting from a single metabolic defect that is best treated by one pharmaceutical agent. In contrast, multi-systemic disease involves a complex array of symptoms involving multiple system defects, and typically requires comprehensive and integrated treatments.

What is integrative medicine?

While advanced surgical treatment is a necessary step in the restoration of health in patients with endometriosis, it does not necessarily address the underlying interplay between environmental, genetic, and epigenetic factors. Nor does it address underlying systemic dysfunction that influenced disease expression and which, in turn, has been influenced by the disease process.

Integrative medicine integrates several modalities to treat the whole patient in a personalized fashion. Unlike traditional western medicine, integrative medicine focuses on patient health, not mere disease management. This means not only having an interest in the absence of disease in the patient, but also in optimizing how all the underlying systems function in the body.

"Evil Siblings" of endo

The "Evil Siblings" of endometriosis can affect multiple systems throughout the body and show considerable symptom overlap. This makes the task of diagnosis and effective treatment challenging. Some conditions are chronic in nature and do not have a definitive treatment. In these cases, management of symptoms and efforts to improve overall health and function may be of the most benefit.

Uterine conditions

Uterine anomalies, fibroids, and adenomyosis are more common in women with endometriosis. Uterine anomalies (abnormalities in how the uterus developed) can affect a woman's ability to carry a baby and may increase the risk of complications during pregnancy and childbirth. Fibroids and adenomyosis may cause excessive vaginal bleeding and/or uterine pain. Adenomyosis is particularly common in women with endometriosis, with some studies reporting up to a 70% overlap between the two conditions. Surgically removing endometriosis will not resolve any uterine problems the woman may also have.

Wicked Womb

Fibromyalgia & chronic fatigue

Fibromyalgia and chronic fatigue syndrome have been found to be more common in women with endometriosis. Both conditions are characterized by fatigue and debilitating symptoms, affecting multiple systems throughout the body. There are no definitive treatments for these conditions, although lifestyle changes may help.

Endocrine dysfunction

Hypothyroidism (an under-active thyroid gland) has been found to be more common in women with endometriosis and can cause weight gain, joint pain, fatigue, and heart disease. Patients with an under-active thyroid often require medication and monitoring.

Atopic disease

Asthma and allergies have again been found to be more common among women with endometriosis. Removing the endometriosis is unlikely to resolve these co-occurring disorders.

Interstitial Cystitis

Interstitial cystitis (IC), or Painful Bladder Syndrome, is very common in women with endometriosis. The inflammatory process associated with endometriosis may trigger or contribute to inflammation of the bladder. This can lead to urinary urgency, frequency, and bladder pain. While removal of endometriosis may reduce bladder symptoms by reducing inflammation, many patients with IC will require additional treatments to manage their symptoms for example, medications, dietary changes, and in some cases, bladder instillations (medications introduced directly into the bladder).

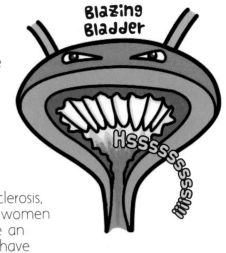

Blazing Bladder

Hsssssssss!!!

Autoimmune disorders

Several autoimmune disorders (lupus, rheumatoid arthritis, multiple sclerosis, and Sjogren's syndrome) have been found to be more common in women with endometriosis. While endometriosis does not itself appear to be an autoimmune disorder and most women with endometriosis do not have co-occurring autoimmune conditions, the disease does have an ongoing inflammatory effect on the immune system. This could result in temporary and/or ongoing systemic effects.

Gastrointestinal disorders

Gastrointestinal and nutritional disorders (such as Irritable Bowel Syndrome - IBS), and food sensitivities and intolerance (such as gluten intolerance), are very common among endometriosis patients. In some cases, the disease is a contributing factor. For example, intestinal endometriosis may present with IBS-like symptoms. In such cases, removal of the disease may resolve or lessen these symptoms. Likewise, adhesions involving the intestines may restrict intestinal motility, resulting in similar symptoms. In many cases, however, surgery may not fully resolve gastrointestinal symptoms (bloating, cramping, nausea, and bouts of diarrhea and constipation). Therefore, other underlying causal factors should be explored and treated. Working with an integrative medicine practitioner and dietitian may help improve gastrointestinal functioning.

BURP!!!

Grizzly Gut

Gurgle!!!

Belch!

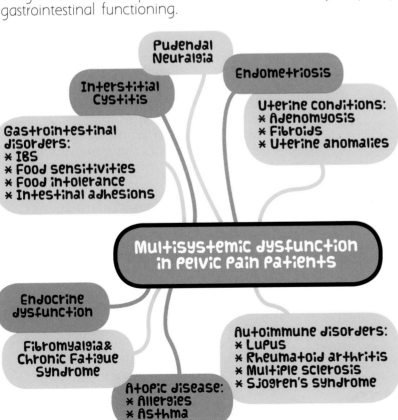

Pudendal Neuralgia

Interstitial Cystitis

Endometriosis

Uterine conditions:
* Adenomyosis
* Fibroids
* Uterine anomalies

Gastrointestinal disorders:
* IBS
* Food sensitivities
* Food intolerance
* Intestinal adhesions

Multisystemic dysfunction in pelvic pain patients

Endocrine dysfunction

Fibromyalgia & Chronic Fatigue Syndrome

Atopic disease:
* Allergies
* Asthma

Autoimmune disorders:
* Lupus
* Rheumatoid arthritis
* Multiple sclerosis
* Sjogren's syndrome

Pudendal neuralgia

Pudendal neuralgia has been found to be extremely common in women with chronic pelvic pain, including those with endometriosis. The pudendal nerve is located along the side of the vagina and has three basic branches: 1) the anterior branch to the clitoris; 2) the middle branch to the vaginal and vulvar area; and 3) the posterior branch to the anus. Pain can be present in any portion of the nerve if it becomes damaged or entrapped, and tenderness may be present in the surrounding tissues. The pain is often worse when the patient is sitting. Pudendal neuralgia can be treated with pudendal nerve blocks and pelvic physical therapy. In some cases, radiofrequency ablation of the pudendal nerve may be helpful.

Domino effects of endo

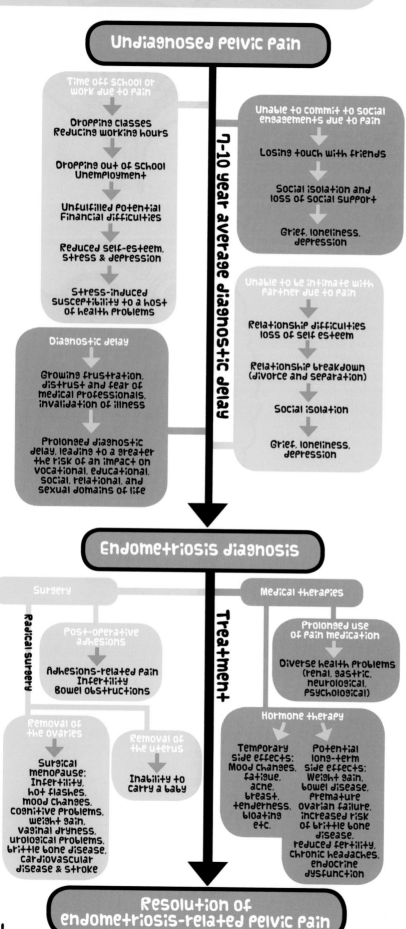

Diagnostic delay & disease mismanagement

With an average diagnostic delay of 7-10 years, most women with endometriosis have endured undiagnosed pain for most of their adult lives. Many have been dismissed as time wasters or told the pain is all in their head. When a correct diagnosis is made, treatment is often inadequate. Patients are often poorly informed of their treatment options. They may be pushed into decisions they would rather not make, such as losing their reproductive organs at a young age or moving forward plans to have a family. These harrowing experiences all have an effect on the individual and her loved ones. The medical trauma so commonly encountered by endometriosis sufferers can continue to haunt a woman even after adequate care has been received. A true healing process must focus on healing both mind and body.

The long-term consequences of medical & surgical therapies

Sometimes one might wonder if the treatments are worse than the disease. Many women endure repeated rounds of hormone therapy, including GnRH-analogues such as Lupron, which induce a temporary state of menopause. Hormone therapies can cause a host of temporary side effects, but there is growing evidence of potentially permanent side effects, including premature ovarian failure, increased risk of osteoporosis (brittle bone disease), reduced fertility, chronic headaches, and an increased risk of inflammatory bowel disease (IBD). In many cases the true long-term risk of hormone therapy is unknown, as it simply hasn't been studied.

Prolonged use of pain medication can result in a host of health problems affecting multiple systems.

Radical surgery (surgery to remove the uterus and ovaries) places a women into an immediate state of premature menopause, bringing with it a host of side-effects and health problems that can affect more or less every system within the body. Any endometriosis surgery carries the risk of post-operative pelvic and abdominal adhesions, but with correct surgical techniques the risk of adhesions is very low.

Ongoing inflammatory disease process

Endometriosis contains cells that secrete irritants that trigger an ongoing inflammatory immune response. The immune system releases inflammatory chemicals called cytokines. Cytokines rush to the site of the disease as well as circulating in the blood stream. This inflammation can result in scar tissue and adhesions, as can the surgery to remove the disease (post-operative adhesions). Adhesions and scar tissue can cause pain, bowel and ureteral obstructions, and infertility. System-wide elevations in cytokines may also cause flu-like symptoms, fatigue, hypersensitivity to pain (hyperalgesia), cytokine-induced depression, and negatively effect adrenal function and cortisol levels (stress hormones). Women with endometriosis have been found to have lower levels of cortisol than women without the condition.

Endometriosis

Endometriotic cells secrete irritants, which trigger the release of inflammatory chemicals by the immune system.

Inflammation (Cytokines)

Systemic increases in cytokines

Scar tissue & Adhesions

Pain

Systemic symptoms:
Flu-like symptoms
Fatigue
Hyperalgesia
Reduced adrenal function
Depression

Bowel & Ureter obstructions

Infertility

Pain

Chronic Pelvic Pain

Reduced Quality of life

Changes in pain perception (Centralized sensitization)

Pelvic Floor Dysfunction

Chronic Pelvic Pain

Chronic pelvic pain can cause a profound reduction in quality of life. It can impact a person's schooling, work, relationships, and sex life. Financial hardship arising from debilitating pain can cause stress and psychological distress, leaving someone more susceptible to depression, anxiety, and a host of physical health problems. Ongoing pain can lead to changes in the way the central and peripheral nervous systems interpret and respond to neutral and painful stimuli. Neutral stimuli may become interpreted as painful, and painful stimuli may evoke even greater sensations of pain (Centralized Sensitization Syndrome - CSS).

Pelvic pain can also result in changes in the pelvic floor muscles. The muscles may tighten and go into spasm in response to pain (Pelvic Floor Dysfunction - PFD), which in turn causes more pain. Even after the original source of pain has resolved, CSS and PFD may continue to negatively impact a patient's life, requiring further treatment.

Understanding underlying risk factors

While it is no woman's fault that she developed endometriosis, it is also true that aspects of our lifestyles and the environment in which we live may influence the onset and course of the disease and its symptoms. Our sensitivity to various environmental factors may be influenced by our genetic make-up. Exposure to these environmental factors may in turn influence gene expression, potentially activating or deactivating genes involved in the onset and course of the disease. Endometriosis risk factors are factors that have been identified as placing an individual at greater risk of being diagnosed with the condition.

While a causal relationship between risk factors and the disease is often difficult to establish, trying to reduce exposure to endometriosis risk factors may influence the disease onset and severity.

The chemicals you ingest and apply to your skin, other sources of environmental toxin exposure, the amount of stress you encounter, the amount of sleep you get, your gut health, and what you eat, all potentially play a role in the course and severity of endometriosis.

The good news is that lifestyle changes potentially provide important ways for you to actively fight this disease over and above traditional treatments.

The truth about toxins...

"Toxins have nothing to do with endo!"
WRONG! Toxins have been linked to both disease incidence and disease severity...

THE EVIDENCE:

1) Dioxin exposure increases incidence & severity of endometriosis: Animal studies and epidemiological studies on humans demonstrate an increased incidence and severity of endometriosis when exposed to toxins such as dioxins, polychlorinated bisphenyls (PCBs), organopesticides, Bisphenol A (BPA), and hormones and antibiotics found in our food supply.

2) Earlier onset of puberty: Girls are reaching puberty at a younger age. We have an increased exposure to environmental pollutants and growth hormones, which may explain the earlier onset of puberty.

3) Dioxins contained in our foods and hygiene products: A major source of dioxins and PCBs is the ingestion of beef, fish, poultry, and dairy products. There are small amounts of dioxins found in tampons and sanitary pads made from rayon or bleached cotton.

4) Organopesticides contained in food: A major source of organopesticides is in fish, meat, dairy, and conventionally grown fruits and vegetables.

5) Dioxins contained in plastics: BPA is found in polycarbonated plastics (such as water bottles and plastic food storage containers) and the linings of canned food containers. These are called xenoestrogens, which increase your total estrogen load.

With the increasing presence of toxins in the food chain, water supply, and household products, there is growing concern about the impact of toxin exposure on our bodies, including risk of developing diseases such as endometriosis.

6) Livestock are fed hormones and antibiotics:
Conventionally raised animals that we consume are given hormones and antibiotics to improve taste and productivity. When we consume these animals, we are getting a low dose of hormones and antibiotics.

7) Heavy metals found in the water supply, foods, and household products:
Heavy metals such as lead, mercury, arsenic, aluminum, and cadmium are found in tap water, large fish, some paints, rice, cookware, deodorants, pesticides, chickens (arsenic is added to their food), arsenic treated wood, amalgam fillings, some toys, glazes on ceramics, and several other sources.

8) Cumulative effect of toxins on cell function:
The bioaccumulation of these toxins in our bodies concentrate in fatty tissues. They interfere with our cells' gene expression leading to detrimental changes in reproduction, endocrine function (hormones), immune abnormalities, altered gut microflora (bacteria in the gut), abnormal growth of cells, and inflammation. All of these changes could lead to increased risk and severity of endometriosis.

Lightening your toxic load

1) Reducing toxins in your diet:
✱ Consume meat/dairy and poultry/eggs from organic, hormone-free, pasture-fed, humanely raised and slaughtered animals
✱ Consume only organic produce. To find out what produce is most heavily sprayed with pesticides go to: www.foodnews.org/pdf/EWG_pesticide.pdf
✱ Drink spring or filtered water

2) Reduce your exposure to environmental toxins:
(Avoid plastics, personal hygiene products, makeup, and smoking) For detailed information on how to reduce environmental toxin exposure visit:
www.ewg.org/consumer-guides

3) Remove amalgam fillings safely:
Look for a dentist who has been trained by the International Academy of Oral Medicine and Toxicology (IAOMT).

4) Increase daily detoxification:
✱ Regular exercise
✱ Sweating
✱ Regular bowel movements
✱ Drinking 1/2 your body weight (lb) in ounces of water
✱ Reducing visceral adipose tissue, the fat in your mid-section (liposuction does not reduce visceral fat! Exercise and a healthy diet does.)
✱ Maintaining a healthy weight and body fat
✱ Diet (we'll come back to that later.)

Stress & Sleep

"What's so important about stress reduction & getting 8-9 hours of sleep?"

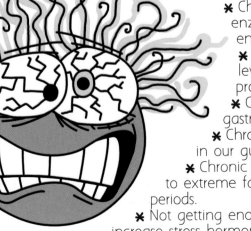

✱ Chronic stress (emotional, physical, or infection) leads to an increase in stress hormones, or our "fight or flight" hormones such as adrenaline and cortisol.
✱ Our stress hormones cause our muscles to be tight (think of overly tight pelvic floor muscles and diaphragm), increase blood pressure, increase blood sugars, and increase inflammation. All of these changes can result in increased pain.
✱ Chronic stress impairs our immune system. Endometriosis is thought to be a condition of immune dysregulation.
✱ Chronic stress increases aromatase activity. Aromatase is the enzyme that produces estrogen. Estrogen can stimulate endometriosis to become more active.
✱ Chronic stress impairs our body's ability to make proper levels of hormones. This may lead to an imbalance in progesterone and estrogen.
✱ Chronic stress impairs our digestion, leading to chronic gastrointestinal discomfort and irregularities.
✱ Chronic stress negatively alters the healthy microbiota balance in our gut.
✱ Chronic stress negatively impacts thyroid function, which can lead to extreme fatigue, weight gain, constipation, insomnia, and painful periods.
✱ Not getting enough sleep (most people require 8-9 hours per night) will increase stress hormones.
✱ Stress reduction may improve pain tolerance and enhance quality of life.

Stress Busters

1) Daily stress reduction: Practice daily stress reduction such as gentle yoga, breathing exercises, meditation, or biofeedback. A great resource is an inexpensive device called heartmath. Learn more at: www.heartmath.com

2) Reset your circadian rhythm: Go to bed at the same time every night (between 9-10 pm), waking at the same time every morning, and going outside without sunglasses for 10 minutes after you wake. Aim for 8-9 hours of sleep.

3) Find positive company: Surround yourself with positive people and people who make you feel good.

4) Avoid negative company: Try to avoid "toxic" relationships that cause stress.

5) Don't overdo it: Do not over-schedule yourself. Learn to say "no" when appropriate and necessary.

6) Love yourself: Cherish and praise your body for what it can do, and show it love and respect. You only get one in this lifetime!

7) Reach out: Don't be afraid to ask for help when you need it!

The gut is just a "food tube" and has nothing to do with endo!

NO!

Endo often goes hand-in-hand with gut problems...

✳ **GI complaints:** GI complaints are common among women with endo.

✳ **Disturbed gut microbiology:** Studies have demonstrated alterations in gut microflora & microbiota in women with endo.

Symptoms: A disruption of gut microflora (dysbiosis) can have negative health consequences, which include impaired digestion, malabsorption of nutrients, increased inflammation (in the gut and systemic), and increased gut infections.

How healthy is YOUR gut?

The role of bacteria in the gut: The bacteria in the gut are involved in proper hormone and neurotransmitter balance, which can alter your moods, sleep, energy, and reproduction.

Consequences: A proper balance in gut microflora is important for estrogen elimination. If gut flora is imbalanced, more estrogen may be re-absorbed. This increases the estrogen load, which in turn can potentially increase disease activity. Healthy gut bacteria are also important for proper digestion and absorption of essential nutrients.

Get your gut into balance

1) Dental hygiene: Brush and floss daily and have regular dental cleanings (remember, the gut starts in the mouth!)

2) Avoid unnecessary antibiotics.

3) Eat fermented foods: Add fermented foods to your diet such as miso, tempeh, fermented vegetables, kombucha, and kefir.

4) Eat fiber: Aim for 25-50 grams of fiber daily to feed your healthy gut bacteria and help to eliminate estrogen. Inulin found in artichokes and onions is especially helpful, as it only feeds your healthy bacteria. Root vegetables, such as winter squashes, beets, and yams, cooked al dente are also yummy for gut bacteria.

5) Take a probiotic if needed: Talk to your health professional about whether probiotics are needed, and if so, which one to take.

6) Test your stool: Have stool testing performed by a specialty lab to evaluate the bacterial balance in your gut. A functional medicine practitioner can help you with this.

7) Avoid sugars and unhealthy fats: Avoid excessive sugar and unhealthy fats, as these feed the unhealthy bacteria.

Should I consider looking into herbal remedies and supplements?

Herbal remedies and supplements can be taken in addition to, or as an alternative, to traditional medications to help reduce inflammation, regulate immune function, modify hormone levels, and repair a damaged gut lining.

How safe are herbal remedies and supplements?

Supplements can be harmful if taken in excess, and in certain cases should only be taken to replenish a deficiency. Some herbal remedies have interactions with prescribed medications, and, therefore, these products should only be taken under the guidance of a qualified healthcare practitioner (such as an integrative medicine practitioner) who is aware of any other medications you may be taking.

Are herbal remedies safer than traditional medications?

While the idea of taking something natural may give rise to the belief that herbal remedies and supplements are always safe, their manufacture is less strictly regulated than that of pharmaceutical drugs. Care needs to be taken when selecting products to ensure their quality and safety. It is also important to remember that many herbal remedies are as powerful as pharmaceutical drugs. Additionally, our bodies use vitamins and minerals synergistically. Adding large amounts of individual nutrients may disrupt this balance. More is not always better!

Just a word on herbs...

The following evidence-based supplements may be helpful:

Pycnogenol: Anti-oxidant, pain reliever.

Resveratrol: Phytoestrogen, anti-oxidant, pain reliever

N-Acetyl Cysteine (NAC): Anti-inflammatory, supports detoxification in the liver (estrogen elimination)

Diindolylmethane (DIM)/Indole-3 Carbinol (I3C): Promotes healthy estrogen breakdown

Magnesium: Important for COMT function (breakdown of estrogen), anti-oxidant, may help with cramping by relaxing the muscles

B vitamins (methylation/conjugation): Important for methylation and conjugation of estrogen (important for estrogen breakdown)

Vit E: Deficiency negatively impacts chytochrome P450 function (detoxification of estrogen) and may lead to elevated estrogen levels, anti-oxidant

Omega-3: Reduces inflammation

Probiotics: Inhibit activity of B-glucuronidase, regulate the immune system, decrease inflammation.

Calcium-D-Glucarate: inhibits B-glucuronidase, increases glucoronidation in the liver (increased estrogen detoxification)

Chrysin: Biflavanoid, inhibits aromatase activity

IMPORTANT! Remember to always work with a qualified healthcare practitioner to determine if you need supplements and to guide you in their safe and effective use.

Food for thought...

Although there is lots of talk about the "endo diet" on the Internet, there is no such thing as a definitive endo diet. There are, however, many common, helpful recommendations that are well supported in the literature. While dietary changes will not make endo go away, they may make living with the disease that much easier. There is no perfect diet for everyone. Diets need to be individualized, based on specific nutritional needs food allergies/sensitivities/intolerance, budget, food preferences, current health status and genetics. This section provides general information only.

Researched foods associated with an increased incidence of endometriosis, worsening of endometriosis-related symptoms, or which are known to alter a healthy balance of hormones (**note:** association does not necessarily mean cause):

Animals raised on grain diets (increase in inflammatory fats = increased inflammation when consumed by humans)

Red meat

Conventionally raised chicken

Animals slaughtered under stressful conditions (increase in stress hormones and inflammatory cytokines = increased inflammation in humans when consumed)

High intake of dairy (increased dioxins and many people are sensitive to dairy, which causes chronic inflammation when consumed)

Farm raised fish (increased environmental toxins & they are often given antibiotics)

Caffeine has been positively associated with endo risk and appears to increase estrogen

A gluten-free diet was shown to significantly reduce pain in 75% of endo sufferers at a 12-month follow up

Alcohol increases estrogen, reduces progesterone, and women who drink alcohol have a higher incidence of endo

A diet high in added sugars and refined carbohydrates raises estrogen levels and increases inflammation

Food sensitivities lead to increased gastro-intestinal & systemic inflammation and gastrointestinal imbalance

Food matters!

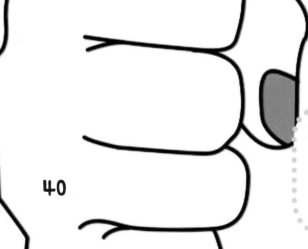

Top tips on beneficial dietary changes for endometriosis...

1) Elimination diet:
Consider a 3-week elimination diet. Continue to eliminate gluten from your diet for 1 year. Consider continuing to avoid or limit dairy even if you are not sensitive to it.

2) Choose your meat & dairy wisely:
Consume meat, dairy, poultry, and eggs from organic, hormone-free, pasture-fed, and humanely raised and slaughtered animals.

3) Be careful with fish:
Consume only small, wild fish in moderation. Consider combining eating seafood with cilantro to help with heavy metal elimination.

4) Go organic:
Consume only organic produce.

5) Drink enough water:
Drink spring or filtered water. Drink half your body weight (in lb) in ounces of water daily to help with detoxification.

6) Avoid alcohol & Caffeine:
Avoid or limit alcohol and caffeine consumption.

7) Low-glycerol diet:
Consume a low-glycemic diet (avoid processed grains such as pastas and breads, overconsumption of fruit, added sugars and sweets, and sweetened beverages).

8) Pescatarian diet:
Consume a highly plant-based, pescatarian diet (fish, whole grains, beans, and lentils, vegetables, nuts and seeds, and fruits).

9) Rainbow diet:
Eat every color of the rainbow in fruits (limit to 1-2 servings) and vegetables (goal is 5-10 servings) daily.

10) Detox:
Consume foods to help enhance detoxification (such as artichoke, cruciferous vegetables, green tea, garlic, pomegranate, onions, watercress).

11) Daily flaxseed:
Consume 3-4 tbsp of ground flaxseed daily to help with the elimination of estrogen and provide healthy omega-3 fatty acids.

12) Root vegetables:
Include root vegetables cooked al dente to provide healthy gut bacteria food.

13) Adequate protein:
Consume adequate protein daily (1-1.5 g/kg of body weight daily).

14) Organic soy:
Consume small amounts of fermented, organic soy if you are not sensitive to soy.

15) Avoid bad fats & oils:
Avoid trans fats, high intakes of saturated fats, and processed oils.

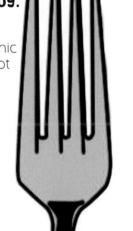

Super foods to help with endo

* **Green tea:** Powerful antioxidant.
* **Lycopene (tomato, guava, watermelon, papaya, grapefruit, sweet red peppers):** Powerful antioxidant; may help reduce adhesion formation.
* **Cruciferous vegetables (broccoli, cauliflower, arugula, radishes):** Help with estrogen metabolism and general detoxification.
* **Turmeric/Curcummin:** Natural COX-2 inhibitor (anti-inflammatory); upregulates detoxification of estrogen and toxins.
* **Flaxseed/Lignans:** Stimulate the production of sex-homone-binding globulin (SHBG) in the liver (reduces free estrogen in circulation); inhibits aromatase activity (reduced estrogen production); fiber binds estrogen in the gut.
* **Fermented foods:** Add healthy bacteria to the gut.
* **Isoflavones (soy, kudzu, clover):** Increase SHBG.
* **Phytoestrogens (soy, legumes, whole grains, flax, seeds):** Bind to estrogen receptor and block estrogen; increase plasma SHBG levels; decrease aromatase activity; shift estrogen metabolism to healthier metabolites.
* **Adequate protein:** Important for formation of digestive enzymes; as inadequate protein intake leads to a decrease in overall cytochrome 450 activity (1st phase of estrogen breakdown).
* **Rosemary:** Improves liver function and promotes healthy estrogen detoxification.
* **Mushrooms (all varieties):** Reduces estrogen production.

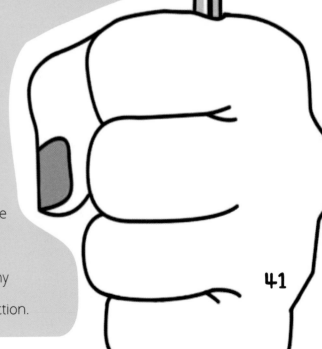

Overview of Supportive treatments & therapies

Pelvic floor physical therapy

Chronic pelvic pain can affect body posture, muscle tone, and alignment. Muscles may become shorter, tighter, and misaligned due to the perpetual responses of the body to pelvic pain. In particular, the pelvic floor muscles may become tighter. In turn, this may contribute to painful intercourse and cause pain and difficulty emptying the bladder and bowel. Pelvic floor physical therapy trains you to relax your entire body, not just the pelvic floor. It helps you to restore balance and alignment. While the pain emanates from the pelvis, the effects of chronic pain can be far-reaching due to the role of the pelvic floor in core activities such as movement and coordination. For this reason, effective physical therapy may need to involve muscle groups throughout the body, including both internal and external work.

Yoga and Pilates

Pelvic floor physical therapy is often combined with gentle exercises, such as yoga and Pilates, to help restore coordination and improve mobility and core strength.

Nutrition & Nutragenomics

Nutrition is the cornerstone of good health. In women with endometriosis, good nutrition can help reduce pain, improve energy, balance blood-sugar levels, address insulin resistance, regulate and improve bowel function, improve your metabolism, control your weight, and positively alter gene expression. The foods you eat have the potential to increase or decrease inflammation and the production of prostaglandins within your body. This may help moderate the painful symptoms of inflammatory diseases such as endometriosis. While dietary changes will not cure endometriosis, they can play an important role in improving overall quality of life.

Nutragenomics is the study of the effects of food on gene expression. Nutragenomics enables us to identify the molecular-level interaction between specific nutrients and dietary components with the genome (the individual's unique genetic code). Nutragenomics provides the exciting potential to offer a truly custom-made nutritional program for the optimization of overall health, based on each patient's unique genetic make-up.

Pain Psychology

Endometriosis is most certainly not "all in your mind", but like any debilitating chronic illness, it has the potential to affect your emotional and psychological wellbeing. Chronic pelvic pain can weigh heavily on your personal, social, and sexual relationships, your schooling or career, as well as on your finances. Simply stated, it can take a tremendous toll on both your mind and your body. Optimal treatment should extend beyond your physical health and include your mental wellbeing and the mind-body connection. Counseling can help you recognize and process the emotional impact of the disease. It can also provide practical coping strategies to help you build resilience, form realistic expectations, and to gradually adjust to a higher level of functioning following successful surgical removal of the disease.

Mindfulness & Meditation

Learning to practice mindfulness and meditation, relaxation, and controlled breathing can help you reduce daily stress. Stress is a major contributor of pain. Enhancing your ability to cope with the physical pain and the emotional burden of endometriosis can greatly improve your quality of life.

...ENDO WARRIOR!... you are an... strong woman with more courage than even you know.... you are a beautiful, intuitive, strong woman r

Hypnotherapy

During hypnosis you are encouraged to enter a mindful, yet trance-like state, rather like day-dreaming. The conscious mind is inhibited and the subconscious mind can be accessed and influenced more directly. In the treatment of chronic pain, progressive relaxation induction (allowing yourself to enter a very relaxed state), distraction techniques, visualization of the pain, and post-hypnotic suggestions for increased resilience and control over pain may be employed. You may also be taught techniques in self-hypnosis to help you relax and cope with pain flares while at home.

Herbs & Supplements

Herbs and supplements can be prescribed as alternatives or in addition to traditional pain medications to lessen the symptoms of endometriosis. They may also be recommended to supplement deficiencies in the body. Talk to a healthcare practitioner with experience in herbs and supplements. They may first want to run tests to determine what you need. Just like traditional medicines, herbal medicines are not without risk. Therefore, it's important to first discuss any herbs or supplements you wish to take with a qualified healthcare practitioner.

Craniosacral therapy

Craniosacral therapy is the use of light touch to manipulate and release restrictions in soft tissue surrounding the central nervous system (CNS - brain and spinal chord). It is believed to help regulate the flow of cerebrospinal fluid. The concept behind the therapy is to restore dysfunction of the CNS, potentially reducing pain, stress, fatigue, backache, and headache.

Acupuncture & Emotional Freedom Technique (EFT)

Acupuncture involves the insertion of fine needles into the skin at specific points of the body. The theory behind the technique is that energy flows through the body along channels (meridians). When these channels become blocked, the body's energy cannot flow freely, and this can manifest in the form of illness. The placement of fine needles at specific points along the body's meridians is thought to allow energy to flow freely once more. This is believed to alleviate symptoms such as chronic pain. While the scientific explanation for the benefits of acupuncture is unclear, it has been speculated that the placement of the needles may stimulate nervous and muscular tissue, providing relief to the patient. EFT or "psychological acupressure" consists of tapping specific acupuncture points on the body, while verbalizing negative emotional experiences. EFT is derived from the belief that negative emotions can play a role in blocking the flow of energy throughout the body. By combining acupressure with verbalization and acknowledgment of negative emotions, balance can be restored to both mind and body.

empty your mind and... allow your body to relax completely... Focus on your breathing.... Focus on the present moment

Body work

Bodywork serves to ease tense and tender muscles, relax your body, and relieve stress. This may help to ease pain and improve your ability to cope. Examples of bodywork include massage (including deep-tissue massage), Reiki, yoga, reflexology, craniosacral therapy, and tai chi. Remember, only continue with a treatment if it helps. If the treatment causes more harm than good, don't do it!

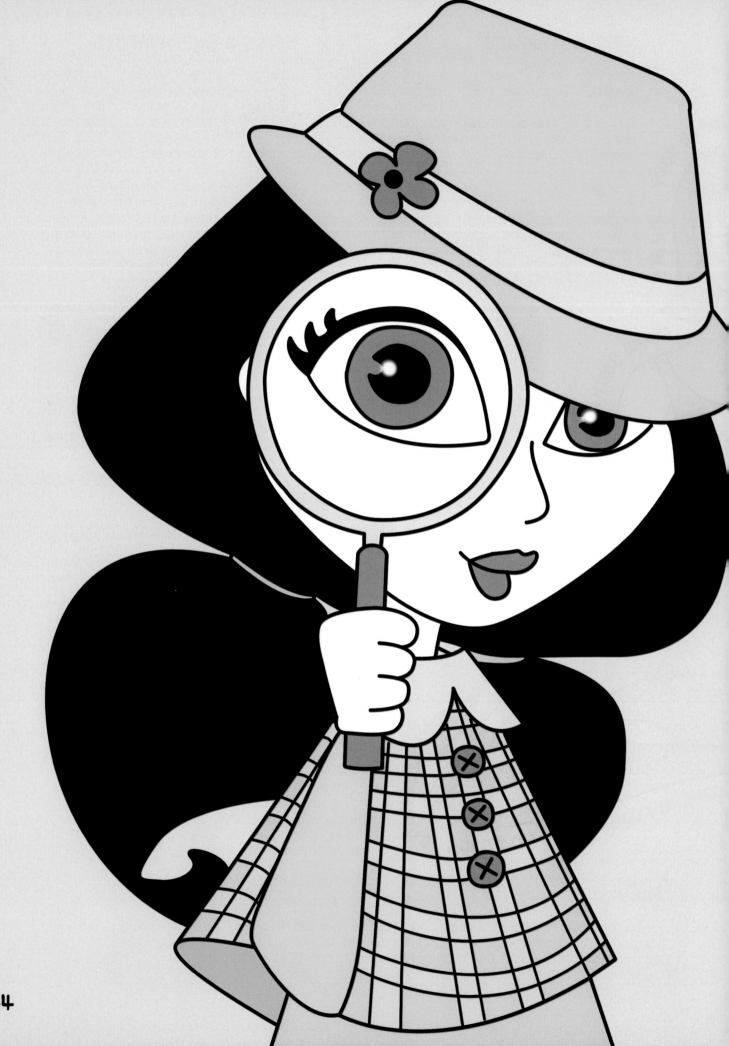

A closer look at:

The endometriosis staging system

Endometriosis and infertility

Endometriosis in teenagers

Endometriomas (chocolate cysts)

Rectovaginal endometriosis

Intestinal endometriosis

Endometriosis and cancer

Adhesions

Endometriosis of the urinary tract

Diaphragmatic endometriosis

What the future holds for endo patients

Adenomyosis

6. Endometriosis Staging

What is the ASRM Endometriosis Staging System?

The American Society of Reproductive Medicine (ASRM) developed a staging system that is commonly used to document endometriosis and associated adhesions involving the uterus, tubes, and ovaries. Patients are classified into one of four stages, ranging from minimal to severe disease.

Given there are **664,381,785,648** possible combinations of point scores within the system, patients within the same stage or even with the same score can vary widely in their disease presentation. For this reason, it is difficult to capture what it exactly means to be categorized as one stage or another, but in general:

Stage 1

Stage 1 disease (minimal disease: **1-5 points**) primarily involves superficial endometriosis (endometriosis limited to the peritoneum, a thin layer of tissue that overlies the pelvic structures). In some cases there may also be small amounts of disease involving the surface of the ovaries and filmy adhesions may be present.

E.9.

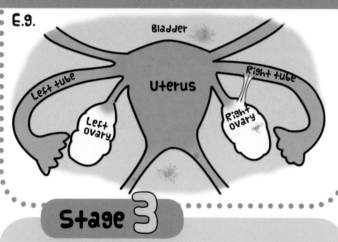

Stage 2

Stage 2 disease (mild disease: **6-15 points**) typically involves more extensive peritoneal disease than with stage 1. Deep disease may be present as may ovarian disease confined to the surface of the ovaries. Again, if adhesions are present, they are likely to be filmy.

E.9.

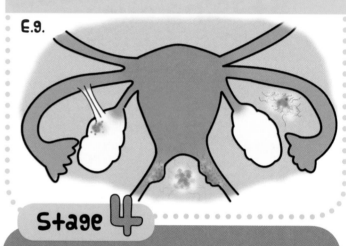

Stage 3

Stage 3 disease (moderate disease: **16-40 points**) may involve small endometrioma cysts inside the ovaries, superficial as well as deep disease (disease that involves the tissue beneath the peritoneum), and is often associated with more extensive adhesions, including dense adhesions.

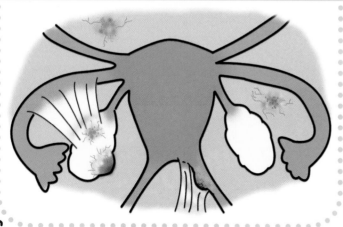

Stage 4

Stage 4 disease (severe disease: **41-150 points**) may involve large endometrioma cysts inside the ovaries, superficial as well as deep disease, and is typically associated with extensive dense adhesions involving the ovaries, tubes, uterus, and bowel, including obliteration of the posterior cul-de-sac (where the uterus has become fused to the rectosigmoid colon).

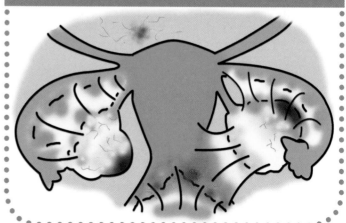

Why do I have so much pain despite only having stage 1 disease?

The staging system does NOT predict pain severity. Women with a higher staging do not necessarily experience more debilitating pain than women with a lower staging. Any stage of endometriosis can be debilitating. The staging system does, however, predict risk of infertility. Patients with stages 3 and 4 are more likely to encounter infertility than patients with stages 1 and 2 disease. This can be explained by the fact that the staging system is weighted toward ovarian disease and adhesions, both of which are leading contributing factors in endometriosis-related infertility. Over half of the points awarded by the system are given for adhesions and not actual disease. Certain forms of endometriosis are not included within the scoring system (including extra-pelvic disease, such as bowel, bladder, and diaphragmatic disease). Likewise, a patient can theoretically have extensive superficial peritoneal endometriosis and still be staged as having "minimal" disease.

Will my disease progress to a higher stage over time?

Stages 1 and 2 disease do not typically progress to stages 3 and 4. Most patients with stages 1 and 2 only have superficial disease confined to the peritoneum. Patients with stages 3 and 4, however, tend to have invasive endometriosis that can involve structures beneath the peritoneum, such as the bowel and bladder. While superficial disease does not seem to become invasive over time, invasive disease may continue to invade more deeply in some cases. Adhesions and scar tissue may also form and worsen over time as a result of inflammation caused by the disease but is most commonly associated with invasive endometriosis.

> **Regardless of stage, early intervention is key in preventing symptom progression.**

7. Endometriosis and Fertility

THE CORE FACTS

1. While endometriosis is a common cause of infertility in women, most patients are still able to conceive and have children.

2. An estimated **30-50%** of women with endometriosis are infertile. Or, said differently, **50-70%** do NOT suffer from infertility (compared to **80%** in a healthy population of women).

3. The likelihood of infertility increases with each stage and is most strongly associated with severe ovarian disease (endometriomas). It is actually still unclear whether superficial peritoneal endometriosis is even linked with fertility.

4. While we have some idea of possible factors that lead to infertility in women with endometriosis, this remains an area of research with more questions than answers.

Are my difficulties in getting pregnant because of my endometriosis?

Not necessarily. There are multiple causes of infertility. While endometriosis is an obvious factor that should be considered, any infertile couple should be evaluated for all possible contributing factors to establish the cause and find a solution if at all possible.

Does having endometriosis mean I won't be able to have children?

No, not necessarily. Most women with endometriosis can have children, either spontaneously or with the help of surgery and/or assisted fertility. Infertility, while common, is not a foregone conclusion in women with this disease.

Should I have children sooner rather than later because of endometriosis?

For any woman, ovarian reserve declines over time. Beyond a given age, a woman's chances of conceiving naturally decline dramatically as she approaches menopause. So, for any woman sooner is better than later, but having children is a big decision and brings up many considerations. While there is no way of knowing what effect endometriosis is having on your fertility now or in the future, you have to make decisions based on your current situation. Remember, most women with endometriosis can conceive and have children, so unless you are planning to undergo surgery that will compromise your fertility (removal of your reproductive organs), there is no reason above and beyond mother nature's biological clock to rush into having children. In cases of very large bilateral ovarian endometriomas, a patient may consider undergoing egg freezing prior to surgery to ensure sufficient eggs are available should she later wish to conceive.

How Might Endometriosis Impact My Fertility?

1 In many cases it does not impact fertility.

2 Inflammatory adhesions involving the ovaries and tubes may prevent the passage of eggs into the tubes, preventing conception.

3 Women with endometriosis have a higher chance of having been born with uterine anomalies (abnormalities of the uterus), which may impact fertility and pregnancy.

4 Radical surgery to treat endometriosis (removal of the uterus & ovaries) will leave you infertile. If you are presented with this option yet still wish to conceive, seek second opinions, and consider undergoing conservative removal of the disease and preservation of your reproductive organs.

5 Other possible causal mechanisms between endometriosis and infertility may well be at play but are yet to be confirmed.

6 Multiple surgeries on the ovaries to treat ovarian endometriomas can reduce ovarian reserve, reducing your chances of becoming pregnant. In most cases, a skilled surgeon can treat the cysts without compromising ovarian function. In fact, removal of the disease has been found to boost fertility.

7 The presence of endometriosis, especially deep endometriosis, can create a "toxic" environment for implantation. The toxic secretions from the endometriotic tissue may potentially interfere with conception.

Does endometriosis pose risks during pregnancy?
No, generally not. Data on adverse outcomes in pregnant women with endometriosis have been mixed. While some studies suggest there is an increased risk of miscarriage, other studies have found no such relationship.

Are there treatments to treat endometriosis-related infertility?
Yes! Multiple studies have found that surgical excision of endometriosis and associated scar tissue can improve fertility rates, especially in patients with severe endometriosis. The key is conservative surgery that fully removes the disease while preserving the reproductive organs. Assisted fertility may also be of benefit to those who cannot conceive naturally, although the chances of fertility treatments being successful improve following conservative excision surgery.

How long after surgery should I wait before trying to conceive and will my chances decline again over time?
While those trying to conceive are most likely to succeed during the first year of trying, this does not mean that improved fertility post-surgery is temporary. The improvements should be ongoing. Essentially, you can begin trying as soon as you feel ready, although generally you are advised to abstain from intercourse for a few weeks following surgery during initial healing.

48

8. Endometriosis in Teenagers

THE CORE FACTS

1. You are NOT alone! Endometriosis is common in teenage girls and is a leading cause of chronic pelvic pain. Up to **70%** of teenage girls who suffer from chronic pelvic pain are later diagnosed with endometriosis.

2. Painful periods are never normal, even in the teenage years. There is no reason why a girl should suffer through this in silence. Your pain needs to be taken seriously and addressed.

3. You aren't too young to have endo, to get diagnosed, or to undergo treatment. Early treatment is key. The sooner this condition is diagnosed and treated, the sooner you can get back to your life as an active teen. A delay in diagnosis and effective treatment can have a devastating effect on a teenager's life. It can impact her schooling, her relationships, and her self-esteem.

4. Just because other women in your family suffer from pelvic pain does not make your pain "normal" or "no big deal". Endometriosis often runs in families, affecting mothers, sisters, and daughters.

Tips for teens

Being a teen isn't easy. It's a time of change, finding your identity, and coping with increasing responsibilities and demands both in and out of school. It's a critical time for learning and development and in many ways, the worst time to have to deal with the onset of chronic, debilitating pain.

Being taken seriously

Many teenagers with endometriosis have a difficult time having their symptoms taken seriously. They are told they're making up excuses, that they're "weaker than other girls", that their pain is normal, or even worse, that it's "all in your head" Of course we know that none of these responses is fair, helpful, or true. The most important thing you can do is to find someone you trust (a parent or family member, teacher, school nurse, pediatrician, or friend) to talk to about your symptoms and to advocate for you in seeking help. If you hit a brick wall, don't resign yourself to silently putting up with this pain. Push for answers, and push for the care you need and deserve. Don't doubt yourself. **YOU KNOW YOUR OWN BODY.**

School and college

Chronic pelvic pain can interfere with every aspect of a teenager's life, including her schooling. If you are missing school, sports, and exams because of pain, it would be helpful to set up a meeting with your school to discuss ways in which they can help you meet your academic goals. This may mean making allowances and adapting your schedule around your most painful days (sitting an exam earlier or later so as not to coincide with your period) or offering extra support to help you catch up on missed work. It may be as simple as providing a quiet place for you to rest and lie down with a heating pad if your pain becomes severe. The more informed your school and teachers are, the better they can help accommodate your needs. There's no shame in speaking up and asking for help. REMEMBER, this is a common condition affecting 1 in 10 teenagers, which means in any given school, plenty of girls are facing the same problems.

Friends and free time

Friends aren't always as understanding as they should be. If you are having to change plans at the last minute because of unexpected pain flares, friendships may be put to the test. Friends may not appreciate how your pain is different from regular menstrual cramps and belittle your situation. After all, it's not always easy to put yourself in the position of another, and often, people base their beliefs on their own personal experiences without realizing that things may be very different for another person. Calmly educating them about your condition and setting out realistic expectations can help avoid disappointment and judgment. If you are worried you may not be feeling up to a night out, perhaps suggest a compromise such as a movie at home, or simply give them a call. Allow your friends to be there for you when you are struggling. Don't shut them out and don't isolate yourself. Having a network of support is essential when dealing with chronic pain.

Going to see the gyn? Dun dun duuuuuuh!!!

Going to see the doctor about your chronic pelvic pain can be a daunting experience, especially for a teenager who has never been to a gynecologist before. You will probably have a lot of questions running through your mind, and you may even be wondering whether it's worth going through such an ordeal in order to get help.

I don't think I can go through with the appointment. How can I possibly talk about such private things with a doctor?

The first thing is to RELAX and BREATHE. It's going to be ok. Every woman goes to see a gynecologist sooner or later. It's just a normal part of growing up and taking care of your reproductive health. While talking to a doctor about topics that are ordinarily considered private and taboo may seem both uncomfortable and unnatural, the truth is that menstruation and sexual health are important topics that are relevant to each and every woman. Said simply, there really is nothing to be ashamed about in talking openly about these topics with your doctor. Your doctor isn't going to be fazed or shocked by anything you have to say. Gynecologists discuss these topics with their patients on a daily basis. It's a normal part of their daily work. They aren't there to judge. They're there to listen and help.

What kind of questions will the doctor ask me? What if I'm too embarrassed to answer them?

The doctor will ask you about your menstrual cycle, whether you are sexually active, and specifically about the symptoms you have been experiencing. It may feel embarrassing to discuss these private topics with your doctor, especially for the first time, but remember, speaking openly about what's going on is a necessary step in getting help. Your doctor listens to patients talking about these same topics all day long, day in, day out. If you are worried you can't find your words, write down a list of symptoms in advance to give to your doctor. You may also find it helps to go to the appointment with your parent or a trusted friend who can offer support and help advocate for you.

What if I don't feel comfortable answering a certain question?

If there is a topic you'd rather not talk about, either bring the relevant information with you written down on a piece of paper for your doctor to read, or politely explain that you'd rather not discuss that particular topic at this point. It's ok to set your own boundaries. Remember, the doctor isn't asking these questions to be nosy but is asking in order to find out what he or she needs to know in order to help you. Try to answer any questions as openly and fully as possible.

Will my parent have to be present?

Your parent can accompany you into the appointment or for part of the appointment, if you feel comfortable with that. You can also request to see the doctor without your parent present. It's your choice, and you should choose whatever you feel most comfortable with.

Can I bring a friend with me?

Yes, bringing a friend with you to the doctor's office, or even into the appointment, can help you feel at ease before and during your appointment.

It's normal to get nervous about your first visit to the gynecologist... and while it's not the most fun experience in the world, it almost certainly won't be as bad as you expect, AND its a necessary step to diagnosing and relieving your pain.... WOOHOO!!!

Will the doctor examine me? If so, what will happen during the exam and will it hurt?

Your doctor is likely to examine you during the appointment in order to evaluate your pain. If you are already sexually active, the doctor will likely perform a pelvic exam, a speculum exam, and possibly an ultrasound to check for tenderness, ovarian cysts, and areas of nodular disease. If you are not yet sexually active, the doctor may skip certain aspects of the exam to avoid causing you unnecessary discomfort. Be sure to ask your doctor beforehand what exactly he or she is going to do, and don't be afraid to raise any concerns you may have BEFORE the exam begins. Having your doctor talk through the various steps of the exam before and during can help you feel in control and more relaxed. If you experience any pain at any point during the exam, tell your doctor. Most women with endometriosis will report tenderness during the pelvic exam. Allowing your doctor to gently map out any areas of tenderness can help determine whether endometriosis might be causing your pain. If the exam is too painful for you to tolerate, the doctor will stop immediately. In some cases, teenage patients are examined under sedation or anesthesia (while you are asleep).

I'm going to be way too embarrassed to undergo the exam!

Don't panic! Having a pelvic exam can be embarrassing especially the first time, but your doctor has performed exams many thousands of times, and its just routine for him or her. You'll have a sheet to cover your lower body, and usually the process takes just a few minutes. You can then get dressed. Sometimes it helps to have a friend, parent, or nurse with you to chat to you and hold your hand during the exam. Talking to a trusted female friend or relative about what to expect during the exam can also help ease any fears ahead of your appointment.

If I see a male doctor, will a female be present during the exam?

The exact rules vary depending on where you are in the world, but typically male doctors are accompanied by a female medical assistant or nurse, who will stay with you during the exam. If no accompanying female is present, you are welcome to request a female chaperon to stand in during your exam. You can also have your friend or parent present with you during the exam. Your choice depends on your comfort level and on your personal preferences.

Exam Room

Tips for parents

When your teenage daughter complains of severe pelvic pain, your natural response may be to minimize her problem in the hopes that it will go away on its own. The best thing you can do, however, is listen to her, comfort and validate her when she is in pain, take her symptoms seriously, and advocate for the best care available. While she may be under the care of a pediatrician, generally gynecologists are more knowledgeable about endometriosis and are the best point of call for a teen with debilitating pelvic pain. Even many gynecologists are unaware that teenagers can be afflicted with endometriosis and may be hesitant to offer treatment to younger patients, especially surgery. If you encounter this, please persist in pursuing a diagnosis and adequate treatment for your daughter. Remember, this can be a very debilitating disease if left undiagnosed and untreated. Early diagnosis and effective treatment are key to resolving the disease, restoring function, preserving fertility, and restoring quality of life. The teen years are critical. Picking up on possible endometriosis at an early age provides the best chance for optimal outcomes for your daughter. With the range of treatments now available, including advanced surgical excision, there's every reason for teenagers diagnosed with endometriosis to live full and happy lives despite this disease.

9. Endometriosis & Cancer

Is there a link between endometriosis and cancer?

Yes, a link has been found between endometriosis and certain rare forms of ovarian cancer (clear cell, endometrioid, and low-grade serous.) The link appears to be greatest in women with cystic ovarian endometriosis (endometriomas.) Women with endometriosis have a 27-80% increased risk of developing these ovarian cancers. While this may seem alarming, this equates to an overall lifetime risk of just 1.5% of developing any form of ovarian cancer (compared to 1% in women who do not have endometriosis.) The vast majority of women with endometriosis never develop a cancer that is linked to their disease, and medications commonly used by women with endometriosis (oral contraceptives and aspirin) have actually been found to decrease the risk of ovarian cancer.

Does endometriosis cause cancer?

We don't actually know how endometriosis is linked with certain ovarian cancers. It could be that there is a causal link, but it can also be that endometriosis simply shares some of the same underlying risk factors for these cancers. Additionally, the risk may be mediated by some of the treatments commonly used to manage endometriosis. A recent Swedish study found that excising endometriosis reduces the lifetime risk of developing these rare ovarian cancers, suggesting that endometriosis itself plays a potential causal role of some kind.

While it is important to keep things in perspective. If you are worried, talk to your doctor...

Do I need to undergo additional routine cancer screening because of my endometriosis diagnosis?

No, while there is a link between endometriosis and an increased risk of certain forms of ovarian cancer, the overall risk of developing these cancers is still so small that endometriosis is not a clinically significant risk factor and, therefore, does not warrant extra screening. It is, however, important that when endometriosis is removed during surgery, all biopsies are sent for pathology confirmation of the diagnosis. Endometriosis can present with a range of symptoms, some of which can mask or resemble other health conditions. Sometimes other serious conditions can masquerade as endometriosis, including certain cancers. Remain vigilant of any symptoms, and follow up on any changes in symptoms or new symptoms you may be having. Also, consider adjusting your lifestyle to reduce your cumulative risk. Risk factors such as obesity and tobacco use contribute to your risk of a range of cancers, including ovarian cancer. Therefore, living healthily and quitting smoking can help reduce your risk.

While endometriosis is a risk factor for certain rare forms of ovarian cancer, the life-time risk of developing these cancers is still very small. Having your endometriosis surgically excised, living healthily, and being vigilant about any symptom changes can help reduce this risk.

10. Endometriomas (chocolate cysts)

What are endometriomas?

Endometriomas are a type of ovarian cyst where the cyst wall contains focal areas of endometriosis and the cyst content consists of old, thick blood that resembles chocolate (hence the name "chocolate cysts"). Endometriomas can range in size from a pea to a grapefruit. Most endometriomas remain between 3-5 cm in size. It's unusual for an endometrioma to grow bigger than 10 cm. While endometriomas sometimes seep their content, it is rare for one of these cysts to rupture, because the cyst wall is thick. Women with ovarian endometriosis almost always have disease elsewhere in the pelvis and are at an increased risk of deeply invasive endometriosis, including intestinal disease. Endometriomas are also often associated with adhesions, which can make surgery more challenging. If you have an endometrioma, it's important to find a doctor who has the necessary surgical expertise to treat severe endometriosis.

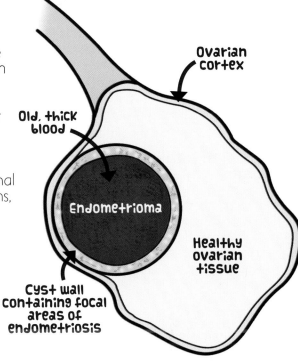

Cross-section of an ovary

Ovarian cortex

Old, thick blood

Endometrioma

Healthy ovarian tissue

Cyst wall containing focal areas of endometriosis

Common symptoms

* Pelvic pain in the area of the ovaries
* Pain during ovulation
* Pain radiating down into the upper thighs
* Occasional attacks of acute pelvic pain if the cyst seeps its content
* Flank pain (if the ovary is stuck to the adjacent pelvic side wall, and presses against the ureter causing back-flow of urine to the kidney)

Diagnosing endometriomas

Enlargement of the ovaries may be detected via pelvic exam. Ultrasound is a highly accurate method of detecting even small endometriomas, but sometimes it is difficult to know whether the cyst is truly an endometrioma or a hemorrhagic cyst (a normal cyst that has bled into itself). While hemorrhagic cysts resolve on their own in time, endometriomas require surgery for their removal. The diagnosis of an endometrioma is confirmed via biopsy following surgical excision (cystectomy).

Treating endometriomas

Surgery is the only way of resolving an endometrioma. **Four** different approaches are commonly used:

Removing the ovary that contains the endometrioma: This can almost always be avoided, if the surgeon is sufficiently skilled. Sometimes an ovary is removed if the patient is already menopausal or if endometriomas keep returning.

Making a hole in the cyst wall and draining the cyst: This approach almost always results in recurrence, because the hole simply heals over and the cyst refills with old blood. Often during emergency surgery, endometriomas are simply drained and the patient soon finds herself back to square one within a matter of weeks. For this reason, planned surgery is preferable.

Draining the cyst and coagulating (burning) the cyst wall: This approach is more effective than simply draining the cyst, but has a recurrence rate of around 20% per endometrioma. Coagulation may not destroy the entire cyst wall and may inadvertently damage healthy ovarian tissue, reducing fertility.

Draining the cyst and removing the cyst wall (excision): This approach has been shown to be the most effective, with a 5% recurrence rate per endometrioma. The ovaries are the site of the pelvis with the highest recurrence rate for endometriosis. This is possibly because small areas of endometriosis may be hidden deep within the ovaries, out of view of the surgeon. Even so, most women with endometriomas do not experience recurrence after excision.

Will Surgical treatment reduce my fertility?

While there is a risk of some healthy ovarian tissue being damaged or removed along with the endometrioma, sufficient ovarian reserve to preserve fertility is almost always retained, provided the surgeon is sufficiently skilled. If a woman has very large endometriomas in both ovaries, she may consider egg-freezing prior to removal of the endometriomas.

Are there any risks in not treating ovarian endometriomas?

Surgery is the only way of treating an endometrioma and formally confirming the diagnosis. Endometriomas usually cause pain and scar tissue. Recent evidence also suggests that endometriomas may cause damage to the ovarian follicles (eggs), and removing an endometrioma may lessen a woman's risk of developing certain rare forms of ovarian cancer. Patient age, future desired fertility, family history, symptoms, and the size of the endometrioma should all be taken into account when deciding what action to take. If an endometrioma is not surgically removed, it should be closely monitored for growth by ultrasound.

Is my endometrioma an emergency?

No, endometriomas are not an emergency. Emergency surgery is best avoided because it may not provide optimal outcomes. It's better to take your time to plan surgery with a surgeon who can manage your case.

If my endometrioma leaks, will it spread endometriosis throughout my pelvis?

Old blood inside an endometrioma may cause acute pain for a few hours or days if it leaks. Leakage may also contribute to adhesion formation. While there is no scientific proof that endometriosis can actually spread when an endometrioma leaks, we cannot be certain that it does not happen.

Will my endometriomas affect my fertility?

Endometriomas may damage the quality of the the ovarian follicles (eggs) and cause ovarian adhesions, inhibiting the passage of eggs along the tubes. Careful surgery to remove ovarian endometriomas and adhesions and preserve healthy ovarian tissue may help improve fertility.

Can small endometriomas be removed?

Very small endomtriomas (under 1 cm in size) may be difficult to find during surgery and tricky to remove, depending on how deep they are.

11. Intestinal Endometriosis

What is intestinal endo?

Intestinal endometriosis refers to disease involving the intestinal tract (the bowel). In most cases it is limited to the serosa or peritoneum overlying the intestines (superficial intestinal endometriosis), but less commonly, it invades into the wall of the intestine (invasive intestinal endometriosis). Intestinal endometriosis affects up to a third of endometriosis patients.

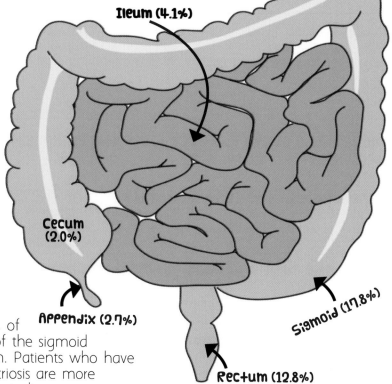

Ileum (4.1%)

Cecum (2.0%)

Appendix (2.7%)

Sigmoid (17.8%)

Rectum (12.8%)

Which parts of the bowel are most commonly affected?

Intestinal endometriosis most commonly affects the rectosigmoid colon. While 17.8% of endometriosis patients have involvement of the sigmoid only 2% have disease involving their cecum. Patients who have more intestinal areas involved by endometriosis are more likely to require bowel resection to treat their disease.

Common symptoms

✖ Pain with bowel movements during menstruation
✖ Pain with bowel movements all month long (invasive disease)
✖ Cyclical rectal bleeding (invasive disease)
✖ IBS-like symptoms (gassiness, bloating, and bouts of diarrhea and constipation)

Diagnosing intestinal endo

Intestinal endometriosis may be suspected based on your symptoms and if nodular disease is felt during the pelvic exam. Superficial intestinal disease will NOT show up via imaging and cannot be felt during an exam. Invasive intestinal disease may, however, be visualized during an ultrasound, CT, or MRI, although this will depend on where the disease is located, how large the nodule is, and how skilled the radiologist or doctor is in interpreting the images. Colonoscopy rarely detects intestinal endometriosis, because even when the disease is invasive, it rarely involves the full thickness of the bowel wall. The disease invades from the outside of the wall inwards, and colonoscopy only inspects the inside. Even if cyclical rectal bleeding is present, the inside of the bowel may still appear normal. Timing the exam, scan, or colonoscopy during your flow may improve the chances of invasive disease being detected. The best way to assess for intestinal endometriosis is to inspect the area during surgery itself. If your scan or colonoscopy comes back normal, this does NOT exclude the possibility of intestinal endometriosis.

Treating intestinal endo

Four different approaches are commonly used in the surgical treatment of intestinal endometriosis:

Shaving: Superficial disease restricted to the outer layer of the bowel (the serosa) can be shaved off of the bowel.

Discoid resection: Invasive disease involving the muscular and mucosal layers of the bowel wall may be treated by cutting out a disc of bowel wall. The disc may involve partial thickness of the bowel wall or the full thickness, depending on the extent of invasion. After the disc has been removed, the defect in the wall is repaired.

Segmental resection: If multiple nodules of invasive disease involve the same section of bowel or a large nodule is present, it may not be feasible to perform a discoid resection (the hole left behind may be too big to repair). Instead, the whole segment of affected bowel may be removed leaving two loose ends of healthy bowel. These ends are then reconnected (re-anastomosis) via staples or sutures.

Appendectomy: If the appendix is affected, an appendectomy is typically performed to remove it.

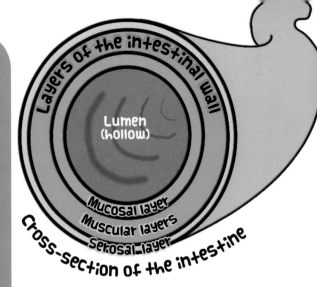

Layers of the intestinal wall

Lumen (hollow)

Mucosal layer
Muscular layers
Serosal layer

Cross-section of the intestine

What are the risks of surgical treatment?

Possible complications include nerve damage resulting in temporary or permanent bladder, bowel, and sexual dysfunction, and post-operative bowel leak. Bowel leaks require emergency reoperation to repair the leak and may result in a need for a temporary or permanent ostomy ("poop bag"). While these are serious complications, in the hands of a highly experienced surgeon, this type of surgery carries low risks of complications. Be sure to ask your surgeon about his or her complication rates.

Are there any risks with not treating intestinal endometriosis?

Generally not, other than persistent pain. There is, however, a small risk of bowel obstruction, particularly in the case of invasive endometriosis of the small intestine, which would present as a medical emergency. There have been a small number of cases of bowel rupture in pregnant women with untreated invasive bowel disease. Again, this is a rare yet serious complication.

Types of bowel resection

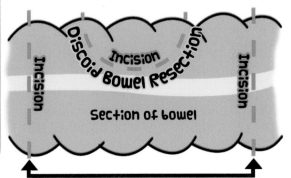

Incision
Incision
Discoid Bowel Resection
Incision
Section of bowel
Segmental bowel resection

12. Urinary Tract Endometriosis

What is urinary tract endo?

Endometriosis of the urinary tract comprises disease involving or overlying the bladder, ureters, and kidneys (the latter of which is extremely rare). Most cases of urinary tract endometriosis involve superficial disease of the bladder serosa (the peritoneum overlying the bladder) and the pelvic sidewalls (which overlie the ureters). Rarely, invasive disease actually invades into the bladder walls (bladder muscularis and bladder mucosa) and/or invades beneath the peritoneum into the space occupied by the ureters. This can potentially constrict the flow of urine from the kidneys to the bladder and cause a build up of fluid inside the kidneys (hydronephrosis). Hydronephrosis resulting from urinary tract endometriosis, while rare, is a serious condition, as it can lead to kidney damage or even kidney failure if the problem is not diagnosed and treated. Most cases of hydronephrosis result from scar tissue associated with invasive endometriosis strangulating the ureter. Very rarely, endometriosis actually invades into the wall of the ureter, causing an obstruction.

Common symptoms

* Urinary urgency and frequency (invasive bladder disease)
* Painful bladder spasm when emptying the bladder (invasive bladder disease)
* Visible or microscopic traces of blood in the urine (invasive bladder disease)
* Bladder symptoms may worsen cyclically
* Symptoms of bladder endometriosis may closely resemble the symptoms of interstitial cystitis (painful bladder symptom), and differential diagnosis may be challenging
* Superficial bladder endometriosis, while a potential source of pelvic pain, does not normally result in specific urinary symptoms
* Flank pain that may worsen cyclically (due to hydronephrosis)

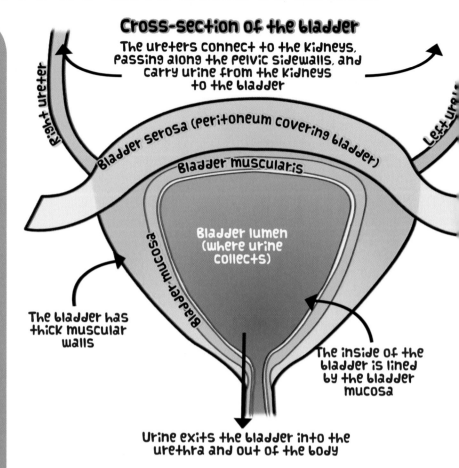

Cross-section of the bladder

The ureters connect to the kidneys, passing along the pelvic sidewalls, and carry urine from the kidneys to the bladder

Right ureter

Left ureter

Bladder serosa (peritoneum covering bladder)

Bladder muscularis

Bladder mucosa

Bladder lumen (where urine collects)

The bladder has thick muscular walls

The inside of the bladder is lined by the bladder mucosa

Urine exits the bladder into the urethra and out of the body

Diagnosing urinary tract endo

Urinary tract endometriosis may be suspected based on a woman's symptoms. Superficial endometriosis of the urinary tract can only be visualized during surgery itself and cannot be seen via imaging. Invasive endometriosis of the bladder wall or pelvic sidewalls may be seen via imaging (ultrasound, CT, or MRI), and may be felt as a mass during pelvic exam. Cystoscopy (a camera inserted inside the bladder), while useful for diagnosing interstitial cystitis, rarely picks up bladder endometriosis because it is very uncommon for disease to invade through the full-thickness of the bladder wall.

Hydronephrosis can be assessed via renal ultrasound, CT scan, and/or IVP (intravenous pyelogram) in which the ureters are checked for constrictions and the kidneys for enlargement. If a constriction is found, a stent (a thin tube) may be placed along the affected ureter to restore the flow of urine from the kidney to the bladder. A full assessment of urinary tract endometriosis may only be possible during laparoscopy.

Treating urinary tract endo

Just as with endometriosis of other areas, the mainstay of the surgical treatment of urinary tract endometriosis is complete excision of all areas of disease followed by repair of any damage to vital structures. Hormone therapy will at best manage symptoms but will not eradicate the disease.

Surgery on the bladder

In the case of the bladder, even if the disease has invaded into the bladder wall, it is possible to cut out the affected area and then repair the bladder wall. In rare cases of full-thickness bladder wall involvement (where the disease invades through the muscular layer and into inner mucosal layer), the patient will need to wear a catheter for a week after surgery to allow for healing. Fortunately, the bladder heals well after this kind of surgery.

Surgery on the ureter

If disease is constricting the ureter, again the area needs to be excised. Usually, the disease and scarring can be removed without cutting into the ureter, but in rare cases, invasion of the wall of the ureter requires ureteral resection (where the affected section of ureter is cut out and the two remaining ends are sutured back together - ureteral re-anastomosis). It is almost always possible to perform this procedure, even if the affected area of ureter is close to the bladder. If ureteral resection is performed, a stent will be placed along the ureter during the surgery and will remain in place for 6 weeks to allow for healing. It is then removed in the office by a urologist. Having a stent can be uncomfortable, but is necessary in order to keep the ureter open and to preserve kidney function.

A note on ureteral reimplantation

Sometimes, if a surgeon is not experienced in treating invasive disease involving the ureter, a urologist will be called in to perform reimplantation of the ureter, often via open surgery. Essentially, the affected area of ureter is bypassed by a section of healthy ureter, which is then reimplanted into the bladder (a psoas hitch) and the nodule of disease is often left in place. While this may provide a temporary solution, the risk is that the section of healthy ureter that has been extended adjacent to the area of disease will later become involved by the same disease process, and the patient will find herself back at square one with recurrent hydronephrosis, yet with fewer options to surgically correct the problem. Furthermore, unless the disease is fully removed, the patient's pelvic pain will very likely persist. It is, therefore, important to find a surgical team that has the necessary expertise to deal with this rare and highly complex form of endometriosis. Discuss your options carefully before consenting to surgery.

What are the risks of surgical treatment?

The main risk of surgery in the area of the ureters is unintentional damage to a ureter. As long as the injury is seen and repaired, the patient will recover. However, if an injury is not seen emergency reoperation may be needed. Likewise, surgery on the bladder carries a low risk of complications, but occasionally a leak may occur at the site of surgery, requiring reoperation. If you are dealing with invasive endometriosis of the urinary tract, it is important to find a surgeon who has the necessary expertise to treat this complex form of endometriosis. Be sure to ask about your surgeon's clinical outcomes and complication rates.

Are there any risks with not treating endometriosis of the urinary tract?

In most cases, no, although persistent pain may worsen with time. However, if a patient has invasive disease constricting or obstructing a ureter, not treating the problem may eventually lead to irreversible kidney damage and kidney failure. In some cases, if a ureteral constriction develops gradually, a kidney may fail without your noticing any symptoms. This is called "silent kidney death".

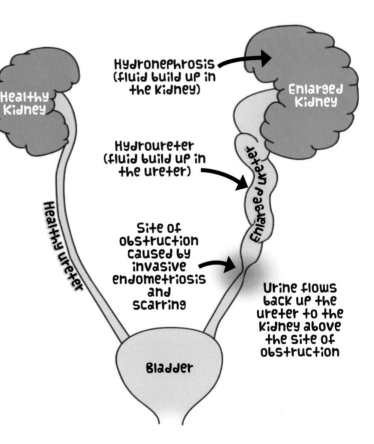

Hydronephrosis due to invasive endometriosis of the pelvic sidewall

Healthy Kidney

Hydronephrosis (fluid build up in the kidney)

Enlarged Kidney

Hydroureter (fluid build up in the ureter)

Healthy ureter

Enlarged ureter

Site of obstruction caused by invasive endometriosis and scarring

Urine flows back up the ureter to the kidney above the site of obstruction

Bladder

13. Rectovaginal Endometriosis

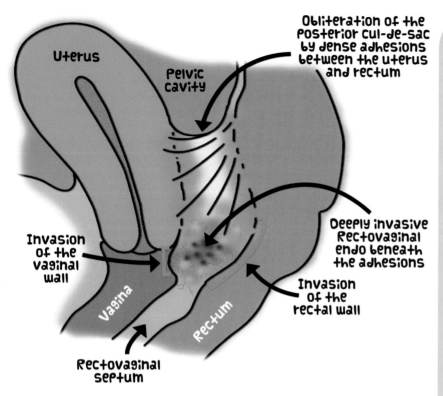

Uterus

Pelvic cavity

Obliteration of the posterior cul-de-sac by dense adhesions between the uterus and rectum

Invasion of the vaginal wall

Deeply invasive Rectovaginal endo beneath the adhesions

Invasion of the rectal wall

Vagina

Rectum

Rectovaginal septum

What is rectovaginal endo?

Rectovaginal endometriosis is a severe form of endometriosis that involves the tissues between the cervix and rectum (the last section of the large intestine). Invasive disease in this area can involve the wall of the rectum, the back wall of the cervix, the uterosacral ligaments (which run between the uterus and the base of the spine), the ureters (which run alongside the uterosacral ligaments), and the inner most portion of the vagina (the vaginal fornix). This form of endometriosis is also commonly associated with severe scarring (fibrosis) in which the pelvic structures have become fused due to the ongoing inflammatory disease process. In such cases, it is not unusual for the uterus to become densely fused to the rectum, obliterating the space between these structures. This is called "obliteration of the posterior cul-de-sac". If the ovaries are also involved by disease, the entire pelvis may be encased in dense adhesions ("frozen pelvis"). With so many important structures in this area, rectovaginal disease often requires very complex surgery for complete removal. The level of skill needed to successfully perform this surgery either requires a surgeon with skills spanning multiple surgical disciplines (gynecology, urology, and colorectology) or a multidisciplinary surgical team that works together on the case.

Common symptoms

Rectovaginal endometriosis can cause severe pelvic pain, especially pain between the vagina and rectum (rectovaginal pain). pain with bowel movements, and deep pain during sexual intercourse (dyspareunia). Women with rectovaginal endometriosis often experience intestinal and urinary tract-related symptoms, depending on which structures are involved. Disease that has invaded through the vaginal wall might also cause a a reddish-pink vaginal discharge, and a tender lump may be felt inside the vagina.

Diagnosing rectovaginal endo

Rectovaginal endometriosis is initially suspected based on symptoms. During the pelvic exam, nodularity may be detected between the uterus and bowel, and if severe adhesions are present, the pelvic organs will be fixed and immobile when palpated. If endometriosis has invaded through the vaginal wall, the disease may be visible during the speculum exam. Ultrasound, CT, and MRI may also detect the disease, although correct diagnosis depends on the skill of the radiologist or doctor interpreting the images. The full extent of the disease will become apparent during surgery, although a surgeon who is inexperienced in treating severe endometriosis may fail to realize that dense adhesions between the uterus and bowel are a sign of underlying invasive rectovaginal disease. Unless the surgeon dissects through the adhesions, the disease hidden beneath may go undetected, resulting in further diagnostic delay.

Treating rectovaginal endo

The key to successful resolution of rectovaginal endometriosis is meticulous surgical excision by a highly specialized endometriosis surgeon. Complete removal may well require the aforementioned techniques used to treat intestinal, ovarian, and urinary tract disease. Furthermore, invasive disease of the vaginal wall can be excised and the wall repaired, restoring sexual function. With the correct surgery, patients with this severe form of endometriosis can expect excellent ongoing relief of their pain.

14. Diaphragmatic Endometriosis

What is diaphragmatic endo?

The diaphragm is a large, flat muscle, shaped like a parachute that separates the chest cavity from the abdominal cavity and plays an essential role in breathing. Very rarely, endometriosis can be found involving the diaphragm. While there have been cases of endometriosis involving both the left and right halves of the diaphragm, the disease is almost always limited to the back portion of the right side. This area is hidden from view behind the liver. Given the diaphragm is thin, invasive diaphragmatic endometriosis is usually full-thickness.

Location of the diaphragm

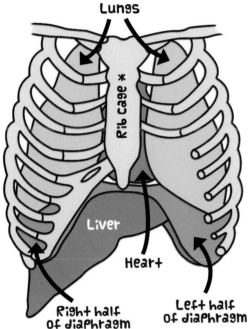

* Some of the left ribs have been partially omitted from the diagram in order to give a better view of the left lung and diaphragm.

What are the risks of surgical treatment?

Surgery on the diaphragm could result in damage to the liver, the lungs, and possible lung collapse. However, in the small number of cases that have been published, few, if any, complications have arisen. If you experience breathlessness or chest pain after surgery, a chest x-ray and thoracic CT scan may be ordered to rule out lung collapse (pneumothorax).

Common symptoms

* Right-sided shoulder-tip pain and chest pain around the time of the menstrual flow
* Pain may radiate up the neck or down the right arm
* Pain may be worse on exercising, breathing in deeply, lying down, and when watching comedy
* In the rare case of left-sided diaphragmatic disease, pain may be present on the left side too

Diagnosing diaphragmatic endo

Generally, diaphragmatic endometriosis is suspected based on the unique set of symptoms and is then diagnosed formally during laparoscopy and biopsy confirmation. Sometimes a mass may be detected via CT or MRI. In order to fully visualize the diaphragm during diagnostic laparoscopy, the liver either needs to be retracted (pulled out of the way) or an extra port needs to be inserted just under the lowest rib margin on the right side. If this does not happen, a portion of the diaphragm will remain concealed behind the liver, and diaphragmatic disease may well be missed.

Treating diaphragmatic endo

The only way of eradicating diaphragmatic endometriosis is to remove it from the body. Hormone therapy and pain medication may be offered to manage symptoms if access to surgery is limited. Disease in this area can be surgically treated in the same way as disease elsewhere, although an extra port just under the ribs may be required in order to access this area. The affected area is removed and any defects to the diaphragm are surgically repaired. A thoracic surgeon may need to be present to assist with excision of diaphragmatic endometriosis.

Are there any risks with not treating diaphragmatic endo?

Diaphragmatic endometriosis is unlikely to present any other adverse effects on your health besides pain, which may worsen over time. In very rare cases, the disease is not limited to the diaphragm but also involves other structures in the chest cavity, such as the lungs, potentially resulting in cyclical lung collapse (catamenial pneumothorax) and bouts of coughing up blood (catamenial hemoptysis).

15. Adenomyosis

What is adenomyosis?

Adenomyosis is a condition in which tissue that somewhat resembles the endometrium is found within the muscular walls of the uterus (the myometrium). Adenomyosis may be scattered diffusely throughout the uterine muscle or concentrated in a mass (an adenomyoma).

Common symptoms

While asymptomatic in some cases, adenomyosis can cause heavy menstrual bleeding, irregular bleeding, and centralized pelvic pain that may refer upwards to the belly button or downwards to the lower back and upper thighs. This is caused by pain being referred along the uterine ligaments. In some cases, surrounding tissues may also be irritated, resulting in bladder and rectal pain. The pain is typically worst during a woman's menstrual flow and ovulation, although pain may be present all month long. Adenomyosis may also be associated with fatigue and a feeling of general malaise that may fluctuate cyclically.

Diagnosing adenomyosis

* **Symptom history:** Adenomyosis is suspected based on your symptoms.
* **Pelvic exam:** An adenomyotic uterus may be tender and enlarged.
* **Imaging:** Ultrasound and MRI are often used to visualize whether nodular or diffuse areas of disease are present within the walls of the uterus. Only in cases of severe adenomyosis will any abnormalities be detected via imaging.
* **Laparoscopy:** Sometimes the outside of the uterus will be abnormal in appearance and consistency, giving rise to a suspicion of adenomyosis.
* **Uterine biopsy:** If an adenomyoma is present, it can be biopsied to confirm the diagnosis. In the case of diffuse adenomyosis, uterine biopsy is rather like searching for a needle in a haystack. The pathologist can only diagnose the disease if an affected area of tissue is contained in the biopsy. For this reason, a negative uterine biopsy cannot exclude the diagnosis.
* **Biopsy confirmation:** Strictly speaking, adenomyosis can only be confirmed via pathology confirmation either via a biopsy or following hysterectomy.

Normal Vs Adenomyotic Uterus

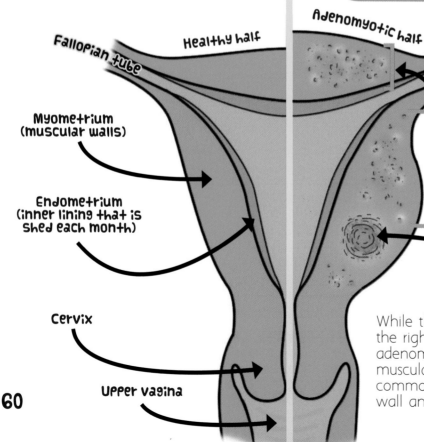

Fallopian tube · Healthy half · Adenomyotic half · Fallopian tube

Myometrium (muscular walls)

Endometrium (inner lining that is shed each month)

Cervix

Upper vagina

Diffuse adenomyosis (disease scattered throughout a large area of uterine muscle)

Adenomyoma (focal adenomyosis - disease concentrated into a nodule)

While the left side of this uterus is healthy, the right side contains both focal and diffuse adenomyosis, causing a thickening of the muscular uterine walls. Adenomyosis most commonly affects the posterior (back) uterine wall and rarely involves the cervix.

My scan was normal. Does that mean I do not have adenomyosis?

No, even with a normal scan, adenomyosis may be present. It may just be too subtle to be detected via imaging. Only advanced adenomyosis is evident via imaging. At the end of the day, the results of an imaging study or biopsy will not change the fact that you have symptoms that need to be addressed. In many cases, adenomyosis will, or should be, suspected and treated based on symptoms alone.

How does adenomyosis impact fertility and pregnancy?

This is a very difficult question to answer. Given the condition usually requires hysterectomy for formal diagnosis and given it commonly co-occurs with endometriosis, it's very hard to research the specific effects of adenomyosis on fertility and pregnancy.

Is there a relationship between endometriosis and adenomyosis?

Yes, while adenomyosis can occur without endometriosis, the two conditions commonly co-occur. Adenomyosis may be especially pervasive in women with deep endometriosis.

Does adenomyosis affect women of all ages?

While adenomyosis is often considered a disease that primarily affects older women, this belief may well have arisen from the fact that the disease is only formally diagnosed after hysterectomy, and younger patients with the condition are less likely to opt for or be offered this procedure. In truth, while adenomyosis may not become symptomatic until a woman reaches her late 20s or 30s, it's a condition that can affect women of all ages, including teenagers.

If you are considering undergoing a hysterectomy to treat your adenomyosis, why not check out www.hystersisters.com for a wealth of information and support!

Treating adenomyosis

Adenomyosis can be treated conservatively (treatment that preserves your uterus) or radically (treatment that removes the uterus). The choice of treatment will depend in part on whether or not you wish to bear children and also on whether conservative treatments are successful in managing your symptoms.

Conservative treatments:

Conservative treatments include hormone therapy, pain management, nutritional supplements, and surgery. Hormone therapy is used to suppress menstruation and reduce estrogen levels, thereby hopefully reducing symptoms. Pain management can also help reduce the pain and inflammation caused by adenomyosis. Nutritional supplements (see pages 44-45) can increase estrogen metabolism and lower estrogen levels, again potentially reducing symptoms. Conservative surgical treatment includes presacral neurectomy (PSN) and adenomyomectomy. During a PSN the nerves that carry pain signals from the uterus to the spine are permanently severed. Even though pain sensations from the uterus are stopped, this procedure may not be completely successful in resolving adenomyosis-related pain. This is because adenomyosis can also cause inflammation in the tissues surrounding the uterus. Adenomyomectomy is where focal adenomyosis (an adenomyoma) is removed from the uterus much like removing a fibroid.

Radical treatment:

If conservative treatments fail to provide sufficient relief, the decision may be made to have the uterus removed (hysterectomy). There are various ways of performing a hysterectomy (vaginally, abdominally, and laparoscopically), and the hysterectomy may be total (the whole uterus is removed) or subtotal/partial/supracervical (the cervix is left behind). The particular technique and procedure offered will depend on the skill set of the surgeon, the patient's medical history, and on her personal preferences. In almost all cases, abdominal (open) hysterectomy can be avoided, provided the surgeon is sufficiently skilled in vaginal and laparoscopic surgery. If you have a history of endometriosis, it is important, to ensure optimal outcomes, that any remaining endometriosis is removed at the same time as the hysterectomy.

Uterine transplants:

A team of surgeons recently succeeded in performing a uterine transplant in a series of women, one of whom became pregnant and delivered a healthy baby boy. There is hope for young women facing hysterectomy for adenomyosis who wish to have children.

61

16. Adhesions

What are adhesions?

Adhesions are bands of scar tissue that have formed between adjacent structures, binding them together. Adhesions can be thin and wispy, like cobwebs, or dense and thick like hardened glue.

What causes them to form?

Adhesions can result from tissue injury, previous surgery, infection, and disease. Endometriosis is a common cause of scarring and adhesions due to the inflammation it causes. Individual differences also play a role; some people are far more susceptible to forming adhesions than others.

What problems can they cause?

Often adhesions cause no symptoms at all. In fact, everyone has physiologically normal attachments, such as those holding the bowel to the abdominal wall. Only when adhesions strangulate or pull on structures do problems occur. If an adhesion pulls on a structure, the patient may complain of sharp, stabbing pains. Intestinal adhesions, for example, may cause pain during digestion and bowel movements, as the bowel expands and contracts (peristalsis), placing adhesions on a stretch. If an adhesion strangulates a structure, serious problems may arise such as obstruction of the ureter or bowel. Obstruction of the ureter can lead to kidney damage, and obstruction of the bowel can require emergency intervention. Adhesions can also affect a woman's fertility, if they involve the ovaries and tubes.

Can post-operative adhesions be prevented?

Various methods can keep adhesions to a minimum:

✱ Performing surgery via laparoscopy rather than laparotomy
✱ Careful surgical technique, such as good control of bleeding, suspending the ovaries away from raw surfaces if they are operated upon and avoiding damage to healthy tissue
✱ Using adhesion barriers (gels, sprays, or sheets) to prevent raw areas from sticking together (Some surgeons have success with using barriers while others find them not to be helpful. Cost is also a factor as some barriers are very expensive and not covered by insurance. It's good to discuss adhesion prevention with your surgeon before your surgery.)
✱ Keeping the number of surgeries to a minimum by removing all endometriosis at the first surgery
✱ Getting up and moving around during initial post-operative healing. Try to not lie in bed all day if at all possible, even if you are only up and about for 10 minutes each hour

How can adhesions be treated?

The primary treatment for symptomatic adhesions is adhesiolysis surgery, in which the adhesions are carefully separated and removed. Successful adhesiolysis requires a highly advanced and specialized surgical skill set, more so than with other types of surgery. This includes gentle tissue handling, keeping the tissue moist, minimal tissue coagulation, meticulous control of bleeding and oozing, and appropriate use of adhesion barriers. In the wrong hands, this complex type of surgery could make matters worse rather than better.

Early Second Look Laparoscopy (ESLL): In patients with very severe adhesions, adhesiolysis is sometimes combined with ESLL. ESLL is usually performed 5-7 days after the first surgery, at which point the adhesions have already formed but have not had time to strengthen. The purpose of the second look is to take down any newly forming adhesions before they become established. Post-operative adhesions form during the first hours and days after surgery. They usually start thin and wispy and become stronger over time. Often adhesion barriers are used to try and prevent adjacent areas of raw tissue from sticking back together. Most patients undergoing endometriosis surgery do NOT require ESLL.

How big a problem are adhesions?

While adhesions can cause severe symptoms, most patients undergoing endometriosis surgery will **NOT** develop post-operative adhesions. In those who do form adhesions, most will not experience any symptoms relating to this scar tissue. The best way to minimize scarring is prevention, and the best prevention is to find a highly skilled surgeon to perform your surgery.

Epilogue

At this point in time, the gold standard of treatment of endometriosis is advanced laparoscopic excision. Meticulous surgery coupled with an integrative, multidisciplinary approach focused on improving overall health not only enables women with this debilitating disease to "survive", but to flourish and thrive in spite of chronic illness. After all, life is so much more than just surviving. We hope that this guide has been of help to you on your journey to a better quality of life.

What does the future hold?

Over the past decades, the number of research articles published on endometriosis has soared. Thousands of studies have been undertaken to try and gain a better understanding of this disease, yet we are still in many ways grappling with the same basic questions. What causes endometriosis? Why does the disease have so many different presentations? Why do some women with endometriosis suffer severe symptoms, while others are seemingly pain free? How can we prevent this disease from developing in the first place? How can we reduce the diagnostic delay? Can we possibly diagnose and treat this disease without the need for surgery? Only time will tell what progress might be made toward answering these questions and accomplishing these goals in the future. There is certainly a momentum underway in pursuit of answers, new avenues of diagnosis, and treatment for future generations of women.

Reducing diagnostic delay

A major problem faced by today's women is a lengthy diagnostic delay. This can set in motion a spiral of decline, affecting all aspects of a woman's life, as she waits for someone, somewhere to take her seriously. Diagnostic delay involves two components: the delay from the time of symptom onset to seeking help, and the delay from seeking help to actually being diagnosed. The normalization of female pelvic pain is a major factor in the intiial delay. Raising awareness about this little-known condition will hopefully prevent future generations of girls and women from suffering in silence. The inadequate amount of training of school nurses, pediatricians, general practitioners/primary care physicians, and OB/GYNs in recognizing and diagnosing endometriosis is another major factor in the diagnostic delay. Continuing education of medical professionals and an expansion of the existing medical school curriculae is desperately needed to provide tomorrow's practitioners more in-depth education on pelvic pain conditions. Too often, it is the patient who ends up searching for answers to explain her ongoing symptoms after not receiving help, rather than her medical professionals volunteering accurate and up-to-date information.

Improving access to care

As we are all aware, diagnosis is only one step in a woman's journey to recovery from endometriosis. Many women find themselves in a never-ending cycle of surgeries and medical therapies without gaining the relief they need in order to function. On the one hand, certain commonly used surgical techniques have been found to leave disease behind in 80-90% of cases, resulting in high rates of disease and symptom recidivism. On the other hand, a small, yet growing community of highly specialized surgeons worldwide are offering their patients complete, wide excision of all areas of endometriosis with minimal rates of disease recurrence/persistence. It is clear that it is time to re-evaluate the mainstay of surgery being offered. Not only do patients need to know about the different types of surgery available but so do their physicians and their health insurance providers. More opportunities need to be provided to train tomorrow's endometriosis surgeons in specialized excision surgery. Recognizing endometriosis surgery as a sub-specialty within gynecology and developing a global surgery accreditation system are important steps toward this goal. Furthermore, the complex and often lengthy surgery required to adequately treat endometriosis needs to be recognized, coded, and reimbursed at an appropriate rate by health insurers. The current situation is both financially unforgiving for the patients and for their surgeons who have spent years mastering some of the most challenging surgery in modern medicine. Only with these provisions can women one day access the gold standard in endometriosis treatment, irrespective of where they live in the world and what financial means they happen to have.

What can I do to effect change?

The only way to bring about change is to spread the word about this disease and the impact it has had on your life. With 178 million sufferers worldwide, it's high time this disease receives the attention and investment it deserves so that the next generation of women need not suffer as previous generations have.

Patient Web Resources

Vital Health's Educational Resources

Patient symptom diary
www.vitalhealth.com/symptom-diary

Endometriosis excision surgery
www.vitalhealth.com/endometriosis-surgery

Pre- and Post-surgery diet
www.vitalhealth.com/pre-surgery-diet
www.vitalhealth.com/post-surgery-diet
www.vitalhealth.com/surgery-diet-faqs

Endometriosis and pelvic pain factsheets
www.vitalhealth.com/patient-factsheets

Endometriosis and pelvic pain blog
www.vitalhealth.com/blog

Surgical videos
www.vitalhealth.com/videos

Patient Support

EndoMetropolis
www.facebook.com/groups/endometropolis/

Endo Warriors
endowarriorssupport.com/

International Patient Support Groups
endometriosis.org/support/support-groups/

Raise Awareness

The Endo Challenge
http://www.endochallenge.com/

The WorldWide EndoMarch
http://www.endomarch.org/

Other Educational Resources

Global forum for news and information on endometriosis
www.endometriosis.org

Endometriosis Foundation of America
www.endofound.org

Comprehensive educational resource on endometriosis
www.endopaedia.info

Participate in Research

Vital Health Research & Education Program
www.vitalhealth.com/about/research-program

The Research OutSmarting Endometriosis (ROSE) Project
www.feinsteininstitute.org/rose-research-out-smarts-endometriosis

The End To Endo (Juneau Biosciences) Project
www.endtoendo.com/

Vital Health Institute
www.vitalhealth.com

Index

About the authors

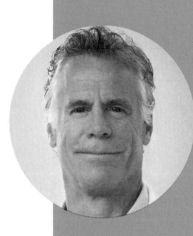

Dr. Andrew S. Cook MD, FACOG

Dr. Cook is a board-cerified gynecologist with a sub-speicalty in reproductive endocrinology, an internationally recognized endometriosis excision surgeon, and a leader in minimally invasive surgery. As Founder and Medical Director of Vital Health Institute in Los Gatos, California, he has been a pioneer in the treatment and management of endometriosis. Known for his compassion, Dr. Cook combines Western medicine and surgical excision with integrative care and a holistic philosophy to help women around the world recover from chronic pelvic pain and return to an optimal quality of life. Dr. Cook started one of the first websites on endometriosis and pelvic pain back in 1996, and he has also authored Amazon Best-seller "Stop Endometriosis & Pelvic Pain" (www.stopendo.com).

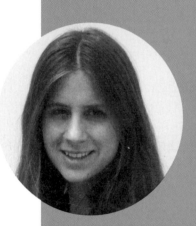

Libby Hopton, MS

Libby coordinates the Vital Health Research Program, a program dedicated to broadening understanding of pelvic pain and endometriosis. She became interested in endometriosis when she was diagnosed with the condition in 2011. As a patient, the quest for optimal treatment felt akin to navigating a minefield of inadequate surgery, ineffective medical therapy, and outright ignorance at the hands of the medical community. The experience motivated her to set up EndoMetropolis and Endopaedia, a large on-line community and web-resource for patients and specialists to discuss and learn about the disease and to advocate for better patient care. Libby's background is in clinical and cognitive neuroscience, statistics and methodology.

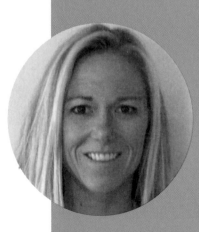

Danielle Cook, MS, RD, CDE

Danielle is Director of the Integrative Specialty Center at Vital Health Institute. She has a Master's Degree in Nutrition and Food Science, is a registered dietitian, and has a diverse background in the field of nutrition, which includes working with women who suffer from endometriosis and chronic pelvic pain. After becoming very ill herself, and failing to get better with traditional (Western Medicine) treatments, Danielle was introduced to Functional Medicine, which in the last eight years, she has studied extensively. She has attended several trainings including the Institute of Functional Medicine's (IFM) Applying Functional Medicine in Clinical Practice (AFMCP), IFM GI Advanced Practice Module, IFM Annual Conference, and The Center for Mind-Body Medicine Mind Body Medicine Training. Danielle is now specializing in functional, preventative medicine and working on her Doctor of Health Science (DHS) in Integrative Healthcare.